Intermittent Fasting and Keto Diet

Smart Guide for Weight Loss, Heal Your Body and Live a Healthier Life; Includes Intermittent Fasting for Women and 28-Day Meal Plan with Quick and Delicious Keto Recipes

ERIC PLAN

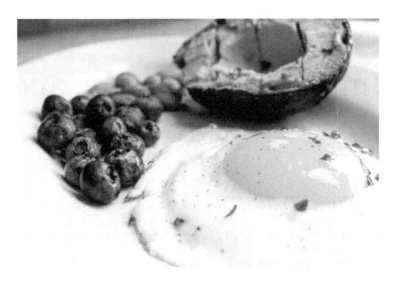

TABLE OF CONTENTS

Introduction

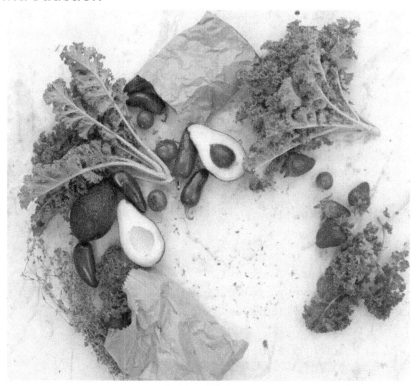

Congratulations on purchasing the *Intermittent Fasting and Keto Diet: Smart Guide for Weight Loss, Heal your body and Live a Healthier Life; Includes Intermittent Fasting for Women and 28-Day Meal Plan With Quick and Delicious Keto Recipes.* Thank you for doing so. Let's begin by learning how the keto plan works with the pyramid!

Basics of Nutrition - The Food Pyramid Explained

Overall: Yes, plenty of water is at the head of the list for every day!

Your Monthly Allotments:

- Four Servings - Red meat

Your Weekly Allotments:

- Three Servings: Eggs - Potatoes - Sweets
- Three to Four Servings: Nuts - Olives - Pulses
- Seven to Fourteen tbsp.: Olive oil
- Four Servings: Legumes - Poultry
- Five to Six Servings: Fish

Your Daily Allotments:

- Three Servings: Fruit - Dairy Products
- Six Servings: Vegetables
- Eight Servings: Non-refined products and cereals (brown rice - whole grain bread - etc.)

Olive Oil: Acts as a major added lipid

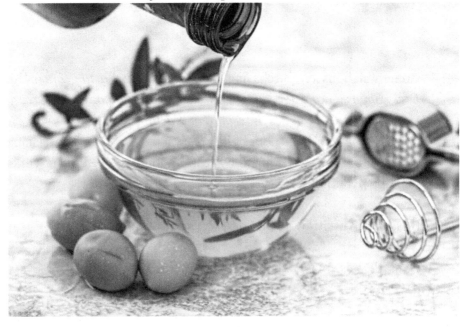

Learn Portion Control

These are some general guidelines so you can better calculate the serving sizes for your meal planning needs:

- Dairy: 1 cup of yogurt or 1 cup of milk / 1.1 ounces of cheese

- Eggs: 1 egg

- Meat: 2.1 ounces of fish or lean meat

- Fruit: 1 orange / 1 apple / 1 banana /1 ounce of grapes / 7.1 ounces of watermelon or other melons

- Potatoes: 3.5 ounces

- Vegetables:1 cup of leafy-raw veggies / .5 cup of all others

- Grains: .5 cup cooked pasta or rice / 1 slice of bread is almost 1 ounce

- Legumes: 100 grams (1 cup) of dry cooked beans

- Nuts: 30 grams (1.1 ounces): Sprinkled on foods for flavor or as a snack

- Wine: 125 ml or about a 4.2-ounce glass of a regular strength red wine

Many benefits will be discussed, including how you can lose and maintain a healthy weight in a sustainable way. Each chapter will carry you through different aspects of the plan and how you can go about changing your eating patterns with the keto diet.

I have filled it with tons of recipes to suit your desires for breakfast, lunch, dinner, and desserts. You are sure to find suggestions to please even the pickiest eater. Before we begin the journey, let's discover how the plan was originated.

The Ketogenic techniques date back in time, as early as the 20th century. The fasting theory was discovered by Bernard McFadden, otherwise known as BernarrMacfadden, as a means for restoring your health. One of his students introduced a treatment for epilepsy using the same plan. In 1912, the *New York Medical Journal* boasted that fasting *is* a successful method to treat epileptic patients, followed by a healthier starch and sugar-free diet.

By 1921, Rollin Woodyatt, an endocrinologist, noted the liver produced the ketone bodies had "three <u>water-soluble compounds</u> including acetone, β-hydroxybutyrate, and acetoacetate" which is a result of a diet highly rich in fats and consisting of low amounts of carbohydrates at the same time.

Also, in 1921, Dr. Russell Wilder, who was employed at the Mayo Clinic, became well-known for the popular ketogenic format. He had a massive interest in the program because he also had epilepsy. The ketogenic methods also became known for its assistance with weight loss and many other ailments.

You will also discover while on the keto diet plan, you will have more energy, and with that energy, you can become more active. Motivation will be the leader as you head toward your new lifestyle making essential changes along the path to success.

After you have the basics, you will enjoy a 28-day menu plan with all of the recipes included. Every item suggested on the plan has the calories, carbohydrates, protein, and total fats listed. It cannot be much easier than this. So, let's Get Started!

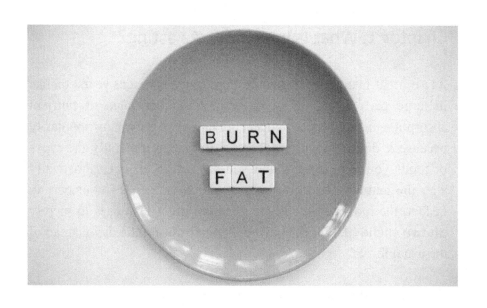

Chapter 1: What Is Intermittent Fasting?

Intermittent fasting has grown in popularity in recent years, thanks in large part to its ability to promote higher rates of nutrient absorption in the meals you eat. It has also grown in popularity because it doesn't require adherents to change radically the types of foods you are eating, when you are eating, or even drastically alter the number of calories you consume in each 24-hour period. In fact, the most common type of intermittent fasting is to merely eat two slightly larger than average meals during the day instead of the usual three.

This makes the intermittent fasting diet plan an ideal choice for those who find they have difficulty sticking to more stringent diet plans, as it only requires changing one habit, the number of meals per day, instead of many habits all at once. Many people find that practicing intermittent fasting leads to real results. It's simple enough to manage successfully over a prolonged period while at the same time being efficient enough to provide the type of results that can keep motivation levels sufficient once the novelty of the new way of eating begins to fade.

The secret to intermittent fasting's success is the simple fact that your body behaves differently in a fasting status versus a fed state. When your body is in what is known as a fed state, it is actively digesting and absorbing food. This begins some five minutes after you have finished putting food into your body and can last anywhere from three to five hours, depending on how complicated the food is for your body to digest. While in the fed state, your body is actively producing insulin, which in turn makes it harder for it to burn fat properly.

The period after digestion has occurred, the insulin levels start dropping back towards normal, which can take anywhere from 8 to

12 hours and is the buffer between the fed and fasted state. Once your insulin levels return to normal, the fasted state begins, which is the period where your body will process fat most effectively. Unfortunately, this means that many people never reach the point where they can burn fat most efficiently, as they rarely go eight hours, much less 12 hours from some type of caloric consumption. There is hope! However, as to start seeing real results, all you need to do is break the three-meal a day habit.

Follow the Golden Rules of Intermittent Fasting as provided within this informative book. You will also discover many new tips and fresh guidelines throughout each segment. In the end, you will know how you can prepare healthy meals while remaining on the fasting protocol using the great recipes provided for you in this book. It's not as hard as you think, as you will soon see. For each of your meals, you can enjoy using your Instant Pot, Crockpot, stovetop, oven, and other conveniences to prepare healthy breakfast, lunch, and dinner meals.

Different Methods of Intermittent Fasting

16/8 Method: The technique is oftentimes referred to as the "lean-gains method" was introduced initially by Martin Berkhan. Its routine targets explicitly your body fat and improves lean muscle mass. One of the most significant benefits of this type of fasting is that it's incredibly flexible so that it will work well if you have a varied schedule. This safe program provides a fasting window of 16 hours, with hours of eating at 8 hours.

This method involves fasting for 14 hours for women compared to 16 hours for men before allowing a reasonable quantity of calories for the remaining 8 to 10 hours. Most people find it helpful to either eat two large meals during the 8 or 10-hour period feeding period or split that time into three smaller meals as that is the way most people are already programmed.

A study was performed by the Obesity Society, stating if you have your dinner before 2:00 p.m., your hunger yearnings will be reduced for the remainder of the day. At the same time, your fat-burning reserves are boosted.

During the fasting period, you should only consume items that have zero calories, including black coffee (a splash of cream is excellent), water, diet soda, and sugar-free gum. The easiest way to attempt this schedule is to stop eating after dinner in the evening and wait 14 hours from there. This means skipping breakfast and picking things up in the early afternoon.

The Warrior Diet: The Warrior Diet was introduced by Ori Hofmekler and takes the 16:8 Program and kicks it up a notch by recommending that you fast for roughly 20 hours out of each day followed by one meal where you get all of your calories in the four remaining hours of the day.

This form of intermittent fasting follows the belief that humans are naturally nocturnal eaters. Therefore, eating at night helps the body better process the nutrients it needs. In this case, fasting is a bit of a misnomer as during the 20-hour period you are allowed to eat a serving of raw vegetables or fruits and maybe a serving of protein if you just can't otherwise continue.

This works because it causes the body's natural sympathetic nervous system to activate a flight or fight response which in turn - increases your natural levels of alertness and increases energy while at the same time increasing the amount of fat burned. The large meal each evening then allows the body to focus on repairing itself and improving its muscles. When following the Warrior Diet, it is important to start each evening meal with vegetables, followed by protein, fat, and carbohydrates used in the keto diet.

This form of fasting is famous for two reasons. First, the fact that a few small and reasonable snacks are allowed during the fasting process, making this type of fasting attractive to those who are attempting the practice for the first time. Second, nearly everyone who tries this form of fasting reports a significant amount of increased energy throughout the day as well as an increase in the amount of fat loss per week.

On the other hand, the relatively strict nature of this diet can make it difficult for some people to follow for long periods of time. The timing of the large meal can also make it difficult for some people to follow because it can naturally interfere with some social engagements. Finally, some people don't like having to eat their food in a specific order. Try it for yourself and see what works for you.

The 5:2 Diet: The plan is also referred to as the "Fast Diet," 5:2 prompts the restriction of calories two days per week to 500 calories daily or two meals at 250 calories while eating normally for five days. It is easy to choose two days to fast and assume your regular caloric intake for the remaining five days. There are not that many statistics on this diet for women, but it is considered safe.

Eat-Stop-Eat - 24-Hour Fast: This technique was initiated by Brad Pilon and requires you to complete a 24-hour fast, but no more than two times in one week. You can select the time you begin the fasting process. Many believe it is easier to fast from 8 pm to 8 pm since so much of the time you will be asleep. You automatically go into ketosis.

When you are finished fasting, it is essential to eat a reasonable or regular diet, and always to avoid binging for an extended period. Fast/binge cycles can cause severe damage to your body. As always, it is important to practice moderation and self-control to get the most out of the fasting cycle.

This fast cycle works on the assumption that to lose a pound of weight each week, all you need to do is give up 3,500 calories. So, it might be best to get it out of the way in two quick bursts rather than fasting for a portion of every single day. This fasting plan emphasizes resistance weight training for maximum benefits.

Going a full day without eating can be difficult for some people at first, but it is perfectly acceptable to work up to a full day of fasting by holding out as long as possible and increasing that amount of time with practice. An excellent way to start is by choosing days that you know don't have any prior food commitments. Beginning a fasting program on a day when you know you have a lunch meeting is just a depraved idea.

When first starting this fast cycle, fatigue, headaches, or feelings of anger or anxiousness are all common side-effects and should be considered a good stopping point for your current fast. These side-effects will diminish as your body adjusts to the news cycle.

After going a full day without any calories, it will be natural to have the desire to binge during your first meal. You must have the self-control to fight these urges since not only is binging bad for you; it can quickly undo all of your hard work from the previous 24 hours. Practice self-discipline and make your fasting worth the effort.

Alternate Day Fasting: This form of intermittent fasting actually means you never have to go long without food if you so choose and is known as the Up Day - Down Day Diet which was created by James Johnson. Every other day you should eat regularly, and on the off-days, you merely consume one-fifth of the calories you normally intake on the average days.

The average daily caloric consumption is between 2,000 and 2,500 calories, which means that the regular off-day varies between 400 and 500 calories. If you enjoy exercising every day, then this form of intermittent fasting may not be for you since you will have to limit your workouts on off-days severely.

When you first start this form of intermittent fasting, the easiest way to make it through the low-calorie days is by trying any one of a variety of protein shakes. It is important to work back to 'real' natural foods these days because they will always be healthier than the shakes.

This form of intermittent fasting is all about losing weight. Those who try it tend to average between two and three pounds lost per week. If you attempt the Alternate Day Diet, it is critical to eat regularly on your full-calorie days. Binging will not only negate any progress you have made, but it can also cause severe damage to your body if continued over time.

Skipping Meals: If you are interested in trying out the benefits of intermittent fasting for yourself, but you have an irregular schedule or are not sure if it is for you, then skipping a meal or two now and then maybe the type of intermittent fasting for you. As previously discussed, getting into a fasting routine is vital to see the maximum results for your effort, but that doesn't mean that fasting doesn't come with some benefits as well.

What's more, once you have tried skipping a meal now and then you can see for yourself just how easy it is, which in turn can lead to more positive changes down the line. With so many intermittent fasting options available, the odds are good that one fits your schedule, so give it a try. What have you got to lose (besides a few pounds)?

Crescendo Method for Women: Dive into fasting without aggravating your hormones or shocking any part of your body using this technique. This is one of the safest programs for women which utilizes a fasting window of 12-16 hours. You can enjoy your meals for 8-12 hours. Space it out for a few days such as Monday, Wednesday, and Friday. If you have failed other diets, this might be your answer. After a two-week time period, add one more day of active fasting to your schedule.

Metabolism and Intermittent Fasting in Women

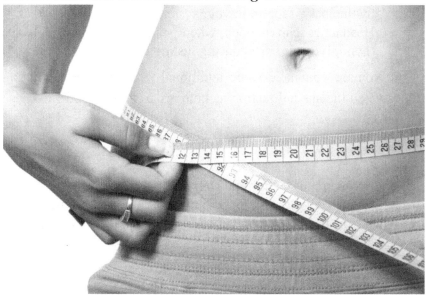

Even with all of the benefits of intermittent fasting techniques, it's unfortunate that women are naturally more sensitive to signs of starvation. This is how it happens. Once your body senses famine - hunger hormones, leptin, and ghrelin - it signals to prompt the hunger.

The leptin is the active hormone that prompts appetite control or the full-satisfied feeling. Once your fast begins, your body stops producing as much leptin. Ghrelin is a hormone that creates a 'hunger' mode. Fasting triggers the ghrelin and makes it rise dramatically. You get hungry, and the cravings begin. It also creates a slowed metabolism rate.

This hormone imbalance can disrupt your hormones and lead to the following issues:

- Depression and Anxiety
- Shrinking of the Ovaries
- Difficulty sleeping
- Fertility issues

- Irregular periods or loss of a period (amenorrhea) caused by the lack of leptin in your system.
- Headaches can happen when your blood glucose levels (hypoglycemia) drop during fasting times.

As a woman, you have some additional stress factors, including times when the special fasting techniques are not a good fit. These are a few:

- When you're nursing
- If you're pregnant
- If you are under chronic stress
- If you struggle with difficulties sleeping or sleep disorders
- If you have a previous food disorder such as anorexia or bulimia

Putting it simply, your body senses the insatiable hunger if you start under-eating. The female's body is actually reacting as if it is protecting a 'potential' fetus - even if you aren't pregnant. Many women ignore the hunger 'cues' and binge later, but the vicious cycle of under-eating can halt ovulation and send your hormones entirely out of whack.

The theory of intermittent fasting was tested for two weeks using female rats. The female indeed stopped having the menstrual cycle, and the ovaries shrunk. They experienced more instances of insomnia than their male counterparts. However, the boys did have lower testosterone production. Even though few human studies portray scientific understanding, but the issues are there.

Are you one of those women who worries about the belly fat and body weight after menopause? If you are, you have the tools at hand to keep those extra bulges under control. Not only that, the intermittent fasting doesn't have an adverse effect on your bones during the aging process. So, ladies chin up and enjoy the fasting techniques used in this diet plan using intermittent fasting.

Back to Scientific Proof

Your metabolic rate is increased with short-term fasting because of the hormonal changes ranging in categories of 3.6% to 14%. Studies have established weight loss after three to twenty-four weeks on the intermittent fasting program to maintain losses of 3.0% to 8.0%. In comparison to other studies on weight loss, these are high percentages that cannot be ignored.

In the same studies, many of the individuals lost 4.0% to 7.0% of his/her waist circumference. This is an indication of how the harmful buildup of belly fat can cause disease and other issues around your organs. You have to consider these results are from eating fewer overall calories, and not binging during the days off. You have to maintain a sensible eating program.

Chapter 2: Intermittent Fasting and the Keto Diet

You will enjoy eating natural foods. The keto diet is low in sugar and processed foods. You can certainly appreciate a diet or a way of life that is close to nature, especially if you can locate some locally produced organic sources.

You will drop the pounds using healthier practices. Your search is over if you are seeking a plan that is worthwhile. The Ketogenic Plan, as it is sometimes called, has been proven to work for weight loss easily and naturally with its many nutrient-dense foods. The focus is placed on healthy fats to keep the carbs moderately low and improve high-quality proteins. The healthy fats, protein, and fiber keep you much more satisfied than candy, chips, or cookies. The veggies make up the bulk of the meal by filling your stomach. You will not be hungry an hour after your meal, and you won't receive a spike your blood sugar.

Specific Benefits for Your Health

Other than weight loss, you can receive benefits from intermittent fasting in many different ways. You will live a longer life from achieving an extended fasting state and diverting your energy while improving your biological functions.

Just remember, the plan will not - in any way cause you to starve. The emergency signals transported by your body is merely that—a signal. The fasting state your body is experiencing will diminish once your body adjusts to the diet method of intermittent fasting you choose to take.

These are some of the crucial elements to consider:

Your Brain Health Will Improve Your brain hormone—BDNF—also known as brain-derived "neuro-tropic" factor—is a protein that can aid in the growth of new nerve cells. Fasting is also believed to provide protection against Alzheimer's and Parkinson's disease.

Cancer Possibilities: Studies using animals have suggested intermittent fasting can be beneficial in the prevention of the disease.

Fatty Acid Oxidation Excelled: Your body will burn more fats as energy with the oxidation process and will also provide quick weight loss.

Risk factors for Alzheimer's are reduced. Research has deemed a 40% reduction occurs for those who use the diet plan, and the risk factors associated with Alzheimer's. Dementia can be treated with medication and aided by the Mediterranean plan. You should also consider some additional exercises to slow the process.

Lower Stress Levels Achieved: The cortisol production is lowered.

Improved asthma symptoms are evident from those using the plan. Numerous studies have revealed the antioxidant diet helped children who followed the plan emphasizing the intake of plant-based foods and a lower intake of red meats.

Reduction in Parkinson's risk factors has been observed. The risk of the disease is cut in half because the high levels of antioxidants in the diet prevent oxidative stress, which is the cell-damaging process. Parkinson's disease affects the cells in your brain, which produce dopamine. You may have some issues with gait and speech patterns, tremors, and muscle rigidity issues. The keto diet can help safeguard you from Alzheimer's, which are triggered by thinking, judgment, and memory loss.

Note: Each of these studies is in the early stages. More research needs to be provided using human testing during the fasting process.

Choose the Right Keto Plan

Depending on your circumstances, you may not have the same goals as another individual. These are the four plans to use as a guideline, so you are aware of the different possible levels involved with the ketogenic way of living:

Keto Method # 1: The standard ketogenic diet (SKD) consists of moderate protein, high-fat, and is low in carbs. Generally, this diet is considered a low-carbohydrate (5% average), high-fat (75% average), and moderate protein (20%) diet plan. These are average counts and can vary.

Keto Method # 2: Workout times will call for the targeted keto diet, which is also called TKD. The process consists of adding additional carbohydrates to the diet plan during the times when you are more active. This is popular with sportsmen and women who are much more active.

Keto Method # 3: The cyclical ketogenic diet (CKD) entails a restricted five-day keto diet plan followed by two high-carbohydrate days.

Keto Method 4: This diet phase is comparable to the SKD phase in all aspects, but you will consume more protein. Its ratio is repeatedly noted as maintaining 35% protein, 5% carbs, and 60% fat. (These are average percentages.)

Keto and How It Works

A ketogenic diet will help you reduce your calorie intake to below the volume of calories your body can spend in one day. Therefore, you need to summon the energy which is stored in your fat cells to deliver fuel/energy to your muscles.

The keto diet will help you to limit the volume of carbs you consume. A substantial portion of your daily fuel will come from fat content which is converted to ketones. A noticeable deal of fat burning can be achieved on greater amounts of calories by sustaining food options used with the ketogenic plan. When you have the protein, carbohydrates, and fat ratio monitored by the diet, as shown in this cookbook; you are well on the way to a successful diet strategy.

You will not be over-eating with large portions of protein. You won't eliminate fat or carbs, which make it a useful and safe diet plan for fat loss.

If you take the approach of eating less, without considering your diet—you will be losing essential minerals and vitamins you need daily—which can result in muscle spasms, fatigue, mental fogginess, hunger, headaches, irritability, insomnia, and emotional depression. You can also lose valuable muscle mass; not just the pounds you intended to drop.

By using the low-carb keto plan, you can reduce your carbohydrates, calorie counts, and nurture your body with a suitable amount of water, meat, eggs, fish, veggies, and nuts, as well as high-quality oils which create fat loss minus the unpleasant side effects.

The Internet provides you with several ways to calculate your daily intake of carbs. Try a keto calculator to assist you. Begin your weight loss process by making a habit of checking your levels when you want to know what essentials your body needs during the course of your dieting plan. You will document your personal information, such as height and weight. The Internet calculator will provide you with essential math.

The Process

Ketosis is used to help you drop extra pounds and burn body fat using healthy eating practices. Proteins will fuel your body to burn the fat, which in turn, ketosis will maintain your muscles and make you less hungry.

Your body will remain healthy and work as it should. If you don't consume tons of carbs, your cells will burn away the fat for energy instead. Your body will switch over to ketosis for its energy source as you cut back on your calories and carbs.

Elements of Ketosis: Lipogenesis and Glycogenesis

Two elements that occur when your body doesn't need the glucose:

The Stage of Lipogenesis: If there is a sufficient supply of glycogen in your liver and muscles, any excess is converted to fat and stored.

The Stage of Glycogenesis: The excess of glucose will convert to glycogen and is stored in the muscles and liver. Research indicates that only about half of your energy used daily can be saved as glycogen. When the glycerol and fatty acid molecules are released, the ketogenesis process begins, and acetoacetate is produced. The Acetoacetate is converted to two types of ketone units:

Acetone: This is mostly excreted as waste but can also be metabolized into glucose. This is the reason individuals on a ketogenic diet will experience a distinctive smelly breath.

Beta-Hydroxybutyrate or BHB: Your muscles will convert the acetoacetate into BHB, which will fuel your brain after you have been on the keto diet for a short time. Your body will have no more food (similar to when you are sleeping), making your body burn the fat to create ketones. Once the ketones break down the fats, which generate fatty acids, they will burn-off in the liver through beta-oxidation. Thus, when you no longer have a supply of glycogen or glucose, ketosis begins and will use the consumed/stored fat as energy.

Foods Included in the Intermittent Fasting Plan
Fresh Fruits:

It is essential to eat plenty of fruits while on the ketogenic diet plan. It is much healthier to grab a fruit versus a handful of candy. Enjoy these according to your <u>daily limits</u> of carbohydrates.

These are some of your best options calculated individually:

- Blueberries: 3 grams per ½ cup
- Strawberries: 8 medium-sized are 6 grams
- Blackberries: 4 grams per ½ cup
- Raspberries: 3 grams per ½ cup
- Plum: 1 medium-sized is 7 grams

This collection of keto fruits are 100 grams each for each (3.5 oz.) serving:

- Apples (12)
- Cherries (10)
- Bananas (20)
- Cantaloupe (7)
- Clementine (10)
- Regular Orange (9)
- Grapes (16)
- Lemon (6)
- Coconut meat (6)
- Mango (13)
- Kiwi (12)
- Peaches (8)
- Pears (12)
- Pineapple (12)
- Watermelon (7)

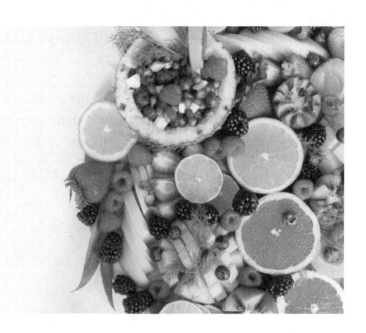

Fresh Vegetables:

Choose from any of these veggies using ½ servings each listed by the Net Carb content:

- Sprouted Alfalfa Seeds (0.2)
- Arugula (2.05)
- Asparagus (6 spears - 2.4)
- Hass Avocado(.5 of 1 - 1.8)
- Bamboo shoots (3)
- Green snap beans (3.6)
- Beet greens (0.63)
- Bell pepper (2.1)
- Broccoli (4.04)
- Savoy cabbage (3)
- Regular size carrots (6.78)
- Baba carrots (5.34)
- Cauliflower (2.97)
- Celery (1.37)
- Chard (2.14)
- Chicory greens (0.7)
- Chives – 1.85)
- Coriander or Cilantro leaves (0.87)
- Cucumber with peel (3.13)
- Eggplant (2.88)
- Garlic (30.96)
- Ginger root (15.77)
- Kale (5.15)
- Leeks – bulb + lower leaf (12.35)
- Red leaf lettuce (1.36)
- Iceberg lettuce (1.77)
- Brown mushrooms (3.7)
- Mustard greens (1.47)
- Yellow onions (7.64)
- Scallions or spring onions (4.74)
- Sweet onions (6.65)
- Banana peppers (1.95)

- Red hot chili peppers (7.31)
- Jalapeno peppers (3.7)
- Sweet green peppers (2.94)
- Sweet red peppers (3.93)
- Sweet yellow peppers (5.42)
- Portabella mushrooms(2.57)
- Pumpkin (6)
- Radishes (1.8)
- Kelp seaweed (8.27)
- Spirulina seaweed (2.02)
- Shiitake mushrooms (4.29)
- Spinach (1.43)
- Crookneck summer squash (2.64)
- Winter acorn squash (8.92)
- Tomatoes (2.69)
- Turnips (4.63)
- Turnip greens (3.93)
- Summer squash (2.6)
- Raw watercress (3.57)
- White mushrooms (2.26)
- Zucchini (1.5)

Special Note for Chili Peppers: The chemical found in chili pepper is called capsaicin which will boost your metabolism. The capsaicin will increase the fat and calories you burn during your intermittent fasting plan. Twenty research studies indicated that you would lose/burn approximately fifty extra calories daily. However, now, all researchers agree with the theory. At any rate, enjoy the chili peppers.

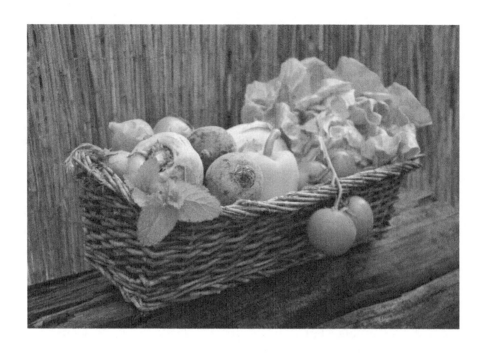

Enjoy Nut Snacks

Each of these options is shown for 3.5 ounces or 100 grams per serving. A rough guideline is approximately three handfuls. These do not include any special toppings such as may be listed as honey roasted, sweet chili, salted caramel, and similar additives. You will consume the carbs quickly as shown:

- 65 pecan halves (4)
- 20 Brazil nuts (4)
- 40 macadamias (5)
- 70 hazelnuts (7)
- 25 walnuts or 50 walnut halves (7)
- 2/3 cup of peanuts (8)
- 80 almonds (9)
- 3/4 cup of pistachios (15)
- 3/4 cup of pine nuts (9)
- 60 cashews (22)

About Almonds: You can grind almonds to prepare almond flour. Its neutral flavor is a superb substitute versus other high-carb flours (more on this later).

Note: These are approximate calculations so you will understand how many portions are in each of the nuts.

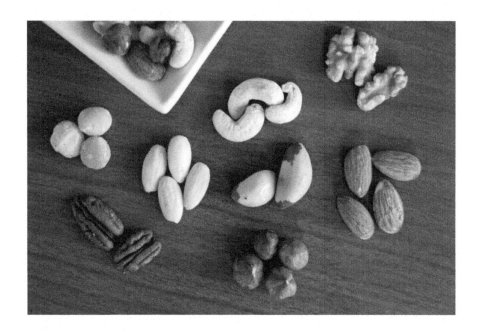

Enjoy Delicious Beverages

Tea: Tea is offered as a good source of beverage because of catechins in the tea conglomerate with the caffeine to help speed up your metabolism. The catechins are an antioxidant and a type of natural phenol which is from the chemical family of flavonoids. An additional 100 calories can be burned daily to increase your metabolism by four to ten percent with the use of green and oolong tea. The effects may be different with each fasting participant.

Coffee: Your caffeine levels can help increase the metabolic rate by approximately 11%-12% to help you remain active when you'd otherwise be tired. Studies have shown the consumption of a minimum of 270 mg of caffeine—about three cups of coffee—will burn away an additional 100 calories daily. The rates can surely boost your intermittent fasting as long as you leave it sugar-free.

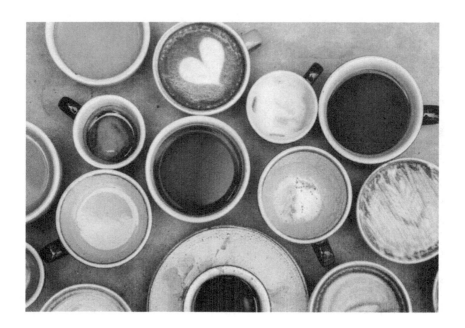

Choose Keto-Friendly Sweeteners

Swerve Granular Sweetener is also an excellent choice as a blend. It's made from non-digestible carbs sourced from starchy root veggies and select fruits. Start with 3/4 of a teaspoon for every one of sugar. Increase the portion of your taste.

Stevia Drops offer delicious flavors, including hazelnut, vanilla, English toffee, and chocolate. Some individuals think the drops are too bitter, so at first, use only three drops to equal one teaspoon of sugar.

Xylitol is at the top of the sugary list as an excellent choice to sweeten your teriyaki and barbecue sauce and teriyaki. Its natural-occurring sugar alcohol has a Glycemic index (GI) standing of 13.

Choose Healthy Fats and Oils

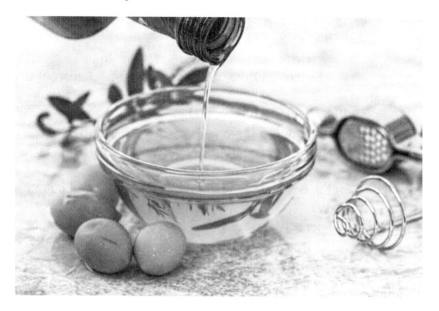

Extra-Virgin Olive Oil (EVOO): Olive oil dates back for centuries – back to where oil was used for anointing kings and priests. High-quality oil with its low-acidity makes the oil maintain a smoke point as high as 410° Fahrenheit. That's higher than most cooking applications call for, making olive oil more heat-stable than many other cooking fats. It contains (2 tsp.) -0- carbs.

Monounsaturated fats, such as the ones in olive oil, are also linked with better blood sugar regulation, including lower fasting glucose, as well as reducing inflammation throughout the body. Olive oil also helps to prevent cardiovascular disease by protecting the integrity of your vascular system and lowering LDL, which is also called the 'bad' cholesterol.

Coconut Oil: You vamp up the fat intake with this high flash-point oil. Enjoy a coconut oil smoothie before your workouts. Use it with your meat dishes, chicken, fish, or on top of veggies. It will quickly transfer from solid form to oil according to its temperature.

Other Monounsaturated and Saturated Fats:

Include <u>these</u> items (listed in grams):

- Avocado, Sesame, Olive, and Flaxseed Oil - 1 tbsp.(0 net carbs)
- Egg yolks – 1 large (0.6 net carbs)
- Olives – 3 jumbo - 5 large or 10 small (1 net carb)
- Unsweetened flaked coconut – 3 tbsp. (2 net carbs)
- Ghee and Unsalted butter – 1 tbsp. (0 net carbs)
- Chicken fat, beef tallow, duck fat, and Organic red palm oil – ex. Nutiva -
  1 tbsp. (0 net carbs)

These are listed so you understand how many carbs can hide in foods you choose while on the ketogenic diet plan.

Stock the Fridge

- *Grass-Fed Butter:* You can promote fat loss and butter is almost carb-free.
  The butter is a naturally occurring fatty acid that is rich in conjugated
  linoleic acid (CLA). It is suitable for maintaining weight loss and retaining
  lean muscle mass.

- *Ghee* is also a great staple for your keto stock, which is also called clarified butter.

- *Yogurt:* Coconut milk is easily digested and contains fats, including lauric acid. Yogurt provides transient bacteria since it feeds existing healthy gut bacteria as they pass through your intestinal tract.

Also, Include These Cold Items:

- Full-fat sour cream
- Goat cheese
- Full-fat cream cheese
- Parmesan cheese
- Hard and Soft cheeses – ex. mozzarella or sharp cheddar

Avoid These Food Items

- *Farm-Raised Salmon:* Much like processed meat, farm-raised salmons are the least healthy type of an otherwise healthy meal choice. When salmon are raised in close proximity to one another for a prolonged period of time, they lose much of their natural vitamin D while picking up traces of PCB, DDT, carcinogens, and bromine.

- *Non-Organic Milk:* Despite being touted as part of a balanced diet; non-organic milk is routinely found to be full of growth hormones. The growth hormones leave behind antibiotics, which in turn, makes it more difficult for the human body to counter infections as well as causing an increased chance of colon cancer, prostate cancer, and breast cancer.

- *Processed Meats:* While protein is an undeniably important part of a healthy diet, seeking your protein from meats, which have been treated, will overload your body full of chemicals. The processed meats tend to be lower in protein while higher in sodium and contain preservatives that can cause a variety of health risks, including asthma and heart disease. Choose from the quality cuts of meat found in most grocery stores.

- *White Flour:* Much like processed meats, by the time white flour has completed the processing, it's utterly devoid of any nutritional value. According to *Care2*, white flour, when consumed as part of a regular diet, has been shown to increase a woman's chance of breast cancer by a shocking 200%.

- *Non-Organic Potatoes:* While the starch and carbohydrates it contains are a vital part of a balanced meal, non-organic potatoes are not worth the trouble. They are treated with chemicals while still in the ground - before being treated again; they are sent to the store to ensure to stay "fresh" as long as possible. These chemicals have been shown to increase the risk of things like congenital disabilities, autism, asthma, learning disabilities, Parkinson's and Alzheimer's disease as well as multiple types of cancer.

Almost "McGriddle" Casserole

Servings Provided: 8
Macro Counts Per Serving:
- **Calories**: 448
- **Protein**: 26 g
- **Fat Content**: 36 g
- **Total Net Carbs**: 3 g

Ingredient List:
- Breakfast sausage (1 lb.)
- Flaxseed meal (.25 cup)
- Almond flour (1 cup)
- Large eggs (10)
- Maple syrup (6 tbsp.)
- Cheese (4 oz.)
- Butter (4 tbsp.)
- Onion (.5 tsp.)
- Garlic powder (.5 tsp.)
- Sage (.25 tsp.)
- *Also Needed*: 9 x 9-inch casserole dish

Prep Technique:
1. Warm up the oven temperature to reach 350° Fahrenheit. Prepare the casserole dish with a sheet of parchment paper.
2. Use the medium heat setting on the stovetop to cook the sausage in a skillet.
3. Add all of the dry ingredients (the cheese also), and stir in the wet ones.
4. Add 4 tablespoons of syrup. Stir and blend well.
5. After the sausage is browned, combine all of the fixings along with the grease.
6. Empty the mix into the casserole dish and drizzle the rest of the syrup on top.

7. Set the timer for 45 to 55 minutes.
8. Transfer to the countertop until it's room temperature.
9. The casserole should be easy to remove by using the edge of the parchment paper. After the casserole has cooled; just slice it into 8 portions.

Bacon Baked Denver Omelet

Servings Provided: 4

Macro Counts Per Serving:
- **Calories**: 345
- **Protein**: 22.4 g
- **Fat Content**: 26.8 g
- **Total Net Carbs**: 3.6g

Ingredient List:
- Butter (2 tbsp.)
- Chopped green bell pepper (.5 of 1)
- Chopped onion (.5 of 1)
- Cooked chopped ham (1 cup)
- Milk - your keto-friendly choice (.25 cup)
- Eggs (8)
- Shredded cheese (.5 cup)
- Black pepper and salt (as desired)

Prep Technique:
1. Program the oven temperature to 400° Fahrenheit.
2. Lightly grease a 10-inch baking dish (round).
3. Prepare a skillet using medium heat temperature setting on the stovetop to melt the butter. Toss in the onion and chopped pepper. Sauté for approximately five minutes. Blend in the ham and cook another five minutes.
4. Beat the milk and eggs in a mixing container. Fold in the ham and cheese mixture. Shake in the pepper and salt. Empty into the casserole dish.
5. Bake about 25 minutes or until the eggs are to the desired consistency.
6. Serve and enjoy.

Bacon Hash

Servings Provided:2

Macro Counts Per Serving:
- **Calories**: 366
- **Protein**: 23 g
- **Fat Content**: 24 g
- **Total Net Carbs**: 9 g

Ingredient List:

- Bacon slices (6)
- Small onion (1)
- Small green pepper (1)
- Jalapenos (2)
- Eggs (4)

Prep Technique:
1. Chop the bacon into chunks using a food processor. Set aside for now.
2. Slice the peppers and onions into thin strips and dice the jalapenos as small as possible.
3. Warm a skillet and fry the veggies.
4. Once browned, combine the fixings and cook until crispy.
5. Place on a serving dish with the eggs.

Banana Avocado Muffins

Servings Provided: 6

Macro Counts Per Serving:
- **Calories**: 332
- **Protein**: 8 g
- **Fat Content**: 30 g
- **Total Net Carbs**: 4 g

Ingredient List:
- Large eggs (3)
- Monk fruit - 30% extract (.25 tsp.)
- Stevia powder extract (.25 tsp.)
- Vanilla extract (1 tsp.)
- Coconut oil (.25 cup)
- Banana extract (2 tsp.)
- Bak. powder (1 tsp.)
- Coconut flour (.25 cup)
- Cinnamon (.5 tsp.)
- Salt (.25 tsp.)
- Almond flour (.75 cup)
- Mashed avocado (1 medium)
- Pecans (.5 cup chopped)
- *Also Needed*: 6-count muffin tin

Prep Technique:
1. Leave the eggs out to become room temperature.
2. Warm the oven to 350° Fahrenheit.
3. Generously grease the muffin tin.
4. Whisk the coconut oil with stevia and monk fruit.
5. Whisk the eggs and mix with the vanilla and banana extracts.
6. In another container, sift or whisk the coconut flour, baking powder, cinnamon, salt, and almond flour.
7. Blend into the coconut oil mixture and the mashed avocado.

8. Fold in the nuts, reserving two tablespoons to sprinkle on top.
9. Empty the batter into the molds and garnish with the nuts.
10. Bake for approximately 25 to 30 minutes.

Blueberry Kefir Smoothie

Servings Provided: 2

Macro Counts Per Serving:
- **Calories**: 476
- **Protein**: 3.9 g
- **Fat Content**: 50 g
- **Total Net Carbs**: 6.6 g

Ingredient List:
- Coconut milk kefir (1.5 cups)
- Fresh or frozen blueberries (.5 cup)
- MCT oil (2 tbsp.)
- Water (+) ice cubes (.5 cup)
- Sugar-free vanilla extract (1-2 tsp.) or pure vanilla powder (.5 tsp.)
- *Optional*: Collagen powder (2 tbsp.)
- *Optional:* Drops of liquid stevia/your choice (3-5 drops)

Prep Technique:
1. Toss all of the ingredients into your blender
2. Pulse until the fixings are well mixed.
3. Serve in chilled glasses.

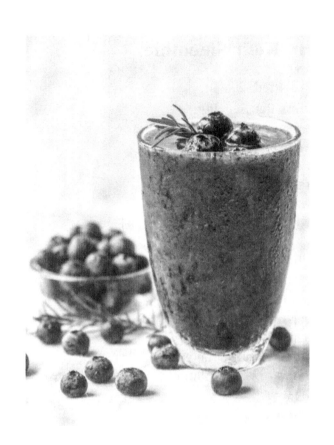

Breakfast Meal-Prep Bombs

Servings Provided: 8

Macro Counts Per Serving:
- **Calories**: 287
- **Protein**: 11.9 g
- **Fat Content**: 24.6g
- **Total Net Carbs**: 2.7 g

Ingredient List:
- Baking soda (.25 tsp.)
- Blanched finely ground almond flour (2 cups)
- Baking powder (2 tsp.)
- Cubed chilled butter (4 tbsp.)
- Sour cream (.33 cup)
- Large egg (1)
- Apple cider vinegar (.5 tsp.)
- Salt (1 pinch)
- Cooked breakfast sausage (6 oz. - crumbled)
- Scrambled eggs (6 large)
- Cooked bacon (4 slices - crumbled)
- Shredded cheddar cheese (.5 cup)
- *Optional*: Sugar-free syrup

Prep Technique:
1. Warm the oven to reach 350° Fahrenheit.
2. Measure and add the almond flour, baking soda, and baking powder in a food processor. Pulse several times to mix.
3. Cube the chilled butter and toss into the processor (low for 20 sec.).
4. Pour the egg, apple cider vinegar, sour cream, and salt to your liking.
5. Let the mixture rest for about five minutes.
6. In a large mixing container, toss the sausage, eggs, bacon, and cheese. Scoop the biscuit mixture into the large bowl. Gently toss to mix with the other ingredients. Using your hands might be helpful.

7. Spray a muffin pan with a spritz of cooking oil spray. Scoop about 1/4 cup of the mixture into each section.
8. Bake until golden brown around the edges (12 to 15 min.). Cool for at least 15 minutes before serving.
9. Store in the refrigerator for up to four days. To reheat, just microwave for 20 to 30 seconds.
10. *Note*: If you use syrup, be sure to add any additional carbs.

Brunch Ham Rolls

Servings Provided: 24

Macro Counts Per Serving:
- **Calories**: 145
- **Protein**: 5.7 g
- **Fat Content**: 9 g
- **Total Net Carbs**: 7.2g

Ingredient List:
- Dried minced onions (2 tbsp.)
- Poppy seeds (2 tbsp.)
- Prepared mustard (1 tbsp.)
- Melted margarine (.5 cup)
- Dinner rolls (24)
- Thinly sliced Swiss cheese (.5 lb.)
- Chopped ham (.5 lb.)

Prep Technique:
1. Set the oven temperature in advance to 325° Fahrenheit.
2. Mix the mustard, onion flakes, margarine, and poppy seeds in a small mixing dish.
3. Make sandwiches using the ham, cheese, and dinner rolls. Place them on a baking sheet. Drizzle the poppy seed mix over the top.
4. Bake until toasted and the cheese has melted (20 min. or so).

Brunch Mackerel and Egg Plate for Brunch

Servings Provided: 2

Macro Counts Per Serving:
- **Calories**: 689
- **Protein**: 35 g
- **Fat Content**: 59 g
- **Total Net Carbs**: 4 g

Ingredient List:
- Eggs (4)
- Butter for frying (2 tbsp.)
- Canned mackerel in tomato sauce (8 oz.)
- Lettuce (2 oz.)
- Red onion (.5 of 1)
- Olive oil (.25 cup)
- Salt and pepper (as desired)

Prep Technique:
1. Warm up the frying pan and prepare your eggs in the butter.
2. Add lettuce to a platter and layer with the onion and mackerel. Place the eggs to the side with a garnish of pepper and salt to your liking.
3. Spritz the oil over the salad and serve.

Carrot Cake Pancakes

Servings Provided: 8

Macro Counts Per Serving:
- **Calories**: 210
- **Protein**: 9 g
- **Fat Content**: 16 g
- **Total Net Carbs**: 5 g

Ingredient List:
- Large eggs (2)
- Unsweetened almond milk (.25 cup)
- Apple cider vinegar (.5 tsp.)
- Coconut flour (2 tbsp.)
- Almond flour (.75 cup)
- Cinnamon (1 tsp.)
- Baking powder (1.5 tsp.)
- Monk fruit erythritol sweetener (3 tbsp.)
- Grated carrots (.33 cup)
- Chopped pecans (2 tbsp.)

Prep Technique:
1. Whisk the almond milk, eggs, and cider vinegar in a mixing bowl.
2. Mix in coconut flour, sweetener, almond flour, baking powder, and cinnamon with a pinch of salt. Whisk smooth.
3. Toss in the carrots and pecans. Set aside while you heat a large skillet using med-low heat.
4. Grease the skillet and spoon the batter in, using about .25 cup per pancake.
5. Cook for 2 to 3 minutes until bubbles form on the edges.
6. Flip the pancakes and cook until they are firm. Place on the serving platter.
7. Continue with the rest of the batter and top as desired.

Cheesy Ham and Chive Soufflé

Servings Provided: 4

Macro Counts Per Serving:

- **Calories**: 460
- **Protein**: 24 g
- **Fat Content**: 38 g
- **Total Net Carbs**: 5 g

Ingredient List:

- Olive oil (2 tbsp.)
- Freshly chopped chives (2 tbsp.)
- Diced yellow onion (1 small)
- Minced garlic (2 cloves)
- Shredded cheddar cheese (1 cup)
- Heavy cream (.5 cup)
- Eggs (6 large)
- Diced ham (6 oz.)
- Salt and pepper (as desired)
- *Also Needed*: 4- 6 oz. ramekins

Prep Technique:

1. Warm the oven to 400° Fahrenheit. Lightly grease the ramekins.
2. Use the medium temperature setting in a skillet on the stovetop to warm the oil.
3. Toss in the onions to sauté for five minutes. Next, toss in the garlic and sauté for one more minute.
4. Whisk together the rest of the fixings in a mixing bowl.
5. Add the cooked onions and garlic. Stir well, then divide among the ramekins.
6. Bake until the egg is done to your liking (18 to 22 minutes).
7. Cool slightly before serving.

Chocolate and Pecan Pie and Muffins

Servings Provided: 12

Macro Counts Per Serving:
- **Calories**: 286
- **Protein**: 4.4 g
- **Fat Content**: 27.1 g
- **Total Net Carbs**: 3.4 g

Ingredient List:
- Swerve Sweetener (.75 cup)
- Pecans - coarsely chopped (1 cup)
- Almond flour (1 cup)
- Salt (1 pinch)
- Softened butter (.5 cup)
- Large eggs (2 unchilled)
- *Optional:* Molasses (1 tbsp.)
- 90% cacao chocolate chopped/sugar-free chocolate chips (2.5 oz.)

Prep Technique:
1. Warm the oven to reach 325° Fahrenheit.
2. Prepare 12 muffins cups with parchment paper liners or silicone liners work best.
3. Whisk the flour, granulated erythritol, salt, and chopped pecans.
4. Beat the butter, eggs, and molasses together until smooth. Whip in the almond flour mixture until just combined. Stir in the chopped chocolate.
5. Dump the batter into the muffin cups.
6. Bake 26 to 28 minutes, or until set.
7. Let the muffins cool in the pan.

Cinnamon Raisin Bagels

Servings Provided: 6

Macro Counts Per Serving:
- **Calories**: 139
- **Protein**: 3 g
- **Fat Content**: 10 g
- **Total Net Carbs**: 6 g

Ingredient List:
- Coconut flour sifted (.33 cup)
- Golden flax meal (1.5 tbsp.)
- Baking soda (.5 tsp.)
- *Optional:* Sea salt (a dash)
- Baking powder (1 tsp.)
- Cinnamon (2 tsp.)
- Whisked eggs (3)
- Apple cider vinegar (1 tsp.)
- Unsweetened coconut or almond milk (.33 cup)
- Melted butter - coconut oil or ghee (2.5 tbsp.)
- Liquid stevia (1 tsp.)
- Golden raisins (.33 cup)
- *Optional*: Vanilla extract (1 tsp.)
- *Also Needed:* Donut/bagel pan

Prep Technique:
1. Warm up the oven to 350° Fahrenheit.
2. Grease the pan.
3. Mix the dry fixings (the golden flax meal, the sifted coconut flour, baking soda, cinnamon, sea salt, and baking powder) thoroughly.
4. In another container, combine the almond/coconut milk, apple cider vinegar, eggs, melted butter/coconut oil, vanilla extract, and stevia.
5. Combine all of the fixings and add to the prepared pan – spreading evenly with a spatula.
6. Bake for 17 to 20 minutes. Cool for three to four minutes.

7. Loosen the bagels with a knife. Turn the bread on the side and slice into half.
8. Serve with toppings of your choice such as butter or cream cheese.
9. Refrigerate or freeze unused portions.

Cinnamon Walnut Flax Muffins

Servings Provided: 12

Macro Counts Per Serving:
- **Calories**: 219
- **Protein**: 6 g
- **Fat Content**: 20 g
- **Total Net Carbs**: 2 g

Ingredient List:
- Ground golden flaxseed or buy flax meal already ground (1 cup)
- Pastured eggs (4)
- Avocado oil or any oil (.5 cup)
- Granulated sweetener - Lakanto coconut sugar, maple sugar erythritol (.5 cup)
- Coconut flour (.25 cup)
- Vanilla extract (2 tsp.)
- Cinnamon (2 tsp.)
- Bak. soda (.5 tsp.)
- Sea salt (1 pinch)
- Lemon juice (1 tsp.)
- *Optional*: Walnuts chopped (1 cup)

Prep Technique:
1. Warm the oven in advance to 325° Fahrenheit. Prepare the muffin tin with paper liners.
2. If starting with whole golden flaxseed, grind it in a coffee grinder, then measure 1 cup.
3. Mix the fixings in the order they are listed using an electric mixer. Add in walnuts *last* after using a mixer.
4. Bake for 18 to 22 minutes. Serve when ready after slightly cooling.

Cream Cheese Coffee Cake

Servings Provided: 8

Macro Counts Per Serving:
- **Calories**: 321
- **Protein**: 13 g
- **Fat Content**: 28 g
- **Total Net Carbs**: 4.2 g

Ingredient List - The Base:
- Eggs (6 separated)
- Cream cheese (6 oz.)
- Erythritol (.25 cup)
- Liquid stevia (.25 tsp.)
- Unflavored protein powder (.25 cup)
- Cream of tartar (.25 tsp.)
- Vanilla extract (2 tsp.)

Ingredient List - The Filling:
- Cinnamon (1 tbsp.)
- Almond flour (1.5 cups)
- Butter (.5 stick)
- Maple Syrup Substitute (.25 cup)
- Erythritol (.25 cup)
- Also Needed: Dark metal cake pan

Prep Technique:

Warm up the oven to 325° Fahrenheit.

1. Separate the egg yolks from whites.
2. Whisk the egg yolks with the erythritol and add with the rest of the fixings. (Omit the egg whites and cream of tartar for the next step.)
3. Whisk the tartar and whites of the eggs to create stiff peaks. Gently work into the yolks.
4. Mix all of the filling fixings to form the dough.
5. Scoop the batter base into the pan. Top it off with half of the cinnamon filling, pushing it down if needed.
6. Bake for another 20 minutes. Transfer to the countertop and top the cake off with the rest of the filling dough.
7. Bake for another 20 minutes to half an hour. Cool for 10 to 20 minutes before serving.

Cream Cheese Pancakes

Servings Provided: 7

Macro Counts Per Serving:
- **Calories**: 149
- **Protein**: 7.2 g
- **Fat Content**: 12.7 g
- **Total Net Carbs**: 0.9 g

Ingredient List:
- Cream cheese (6 oz.)
- Eggs: 4 duck or 6 large hen
- *Optional*: 15 drops vanilla stevia drops
- Whole psyllium husks (1 tbsp.)

Prep Technique:
1. Combine all of the fixings in a processor or small blender.
2. When creamy, add 3 tbsp. of the batter into a frying pan or hot griddle.
3. When it bubbles; just flip and continue browning until done.
4. Garnish with your favorite low-carb toppings.

Egg Muffins - Six-Pack

Servings Provided: 6

Macro Counts Per Serving:
- **Calories**: 148.6
- **Protein**: 11 g
- **Fat Content**: 13 g
- **Total Net Carbs**: 1.1 g

Ingredient List:
- Eggs (6)
- Olive oil (1 tbsp.)
- Diced onion (.25 cup)
- Clove of garlic(1)
- Fresh spinach (2 cups)
- Cheddar cheese - shredded reduced-fat (.75 cup)
- Slices turkey bacon (3 chopped and cooked)
- Milk (1 tbsp.)
- Black Pepper and salt (.5 tsp.)

Prep Technique:
1. Place the oven temperature setting at 350° Fahrenheit.
2. Prepare a sauté pan using the oil.
3. Combine the onion and prepare using the medium heat setting for approximately two mins. Blend the spinach with the onions until it wilts; roughly two or three more minutes.
4. Place the garlic in the pan and continue cooking for 30 seconds. Spice it with pepper and salt.
5. Whip the milk, cheese, and eggs in a separate dish. Toss in the bacon and spinach mixture.
6. Fill the muffin tins about ¾ full.
7. It's ready in 20 minutes or when the muffins are light brown around the edges.
8. Note: You can reheat them for 20 to 30 seconds in the microwave.

Lemon Sour Cream Muffins

Servings Provided: 12

Macro Counts Per Serving:
- **Calories**: 170
- **Protein**: 2 g
- **Fat Content**: 16 g
- **Total Net Carbs**: 3 g

Ingredient List:
- Butter - divided (.75 cup)
- Baking powder (2 tsp.)
- Almond flour - divided (2.25 cups)
- Coconut flour - divided (.5 cup + 1 tbsp.)
- Sour cream - full-fat (1 cup)
- Fresh lemon juice (3 tbsp.)
- Vanilla extract (1 tsp.)
- So Nourished erythritol sweetener - divided (1 cup)
- Xanthan gum (.25 tsp.)
- Lemon zest (1 tsp.)

Prep Technique:
1. Warm the oven to 350° Fahrenheit.
2. Prepare a muffin pan with paper liners.
3. Combine .5 cup butter, .75 cup granulated erythritol, .5 cup coconut flour, 1.5 cups almond flour, sour cream, lemon juice, baking powder, vanilla extract, and xanthan gum in a blender.
4. Mix well until combined, scraping down the sides as needed.
5. Melt the remaining butter then stir in the remaining almond flour, granulated erythritol, and coconut flour.
6. Stir in the lemon zest until it forms a crumbly mixture.
7. Divide the muffin batter among the 12 cups and top each with lemon streusel topping.
8. Bake for 30-35 minutes.

Maple Cinnamon 'Noatmeal'

Servings Provided: 1

Macro Counts Per Serving:
- **Calories**: 376
- **Protein**: 33.7 g
- **Fat Content**: 23.1 g
- **Total Net Carbs**: 4.4 g

Ingredient List:
- Hulled hemp seeds (3 tbsp.)
- Vega Clean Protein in Vanilla (3 tbsp.)
- Ground flax seeds (2 tbsp.)
- Cinnamon (.5 tsp.)
- Lakanto sugar-free maple syrup (2 tbsp.)
- Hot water (.75 cup)

Prep Technique:
1. Combine the dry components in a dish. Whisk and add the water, stirring to thicken as it cools.
2. Top it off with the syrup and serve.

Maple Pumpkin Flaxseed Muffins

Servings Provided: 10

Macro Counts Per Serving:
- **Calories**: 120
- **Protein**: 5 g
- **Fat Content**: 8.5 g
- **Total Net Carbs**: 2 g

Ingredient List:
- Ground flaxseeds (1.25 cups)
- Baking powder (.5 tbsp.)
- Erythritol (.33 cup)
- Cinnamon (1 tbsp.)
- Salt (.5 tsp.)
- Pumpkin pie spice (1 tbsp.)
- Coconut oil (2 tbsp.)
- Pure pumpkin puree (1 cup)
- Egg (1)
- Vanilla extract (.5 tsp.)
- Apple cider vinegar (.5 tsp.)
- Maple syrup (.25 cup)
- *Topping*: Pumpkin seeds
- *Useful*: Blender such as NutriBullet

Prep Technique:
1. Set the oven temperature to 350° Fahrenheit.
2. Prepare a 10-count muffin tin with silicone cupcake liners.
3. Add the seeds to the NutriBullet about one second – no longer or it could become damp.
4. Combine the dry fixings and whisk until well mixed. Add the puree, vanilla extract, and pumpkin spice. Add the maple syrup (1/2 tsp.) if using.
5. Blend in the oil, egg, and vinegar. Combine nuts or any other fold-ins of your choice but add the carbs or calories.

6. Scoop the mixture by the tablespoon into the cupcake liners. Garnish with some of the pumpkin seeds. Leave a little space at the top since they will rise.
7. Bake for approximately 20 minutes. They are ready when they are slightly browned. Let them cool a few minutes and add some ghee/butter.

Mexican Breakfast Casserole – Crockpot

Servings Provided: 10

Macro Counts Per Serving:
- **Calories**: 320
- **Protein**: 17.9 g
- **Fat Content**: 24.1 g
- **Total Net Carbs**: 5.2 g

Ingredient List:
- Pork sausage roll (12 oz. pkg.)
- Chili powder (1 tsp.)
- Coriander (.5 tsp.)
- Garlic powder (.5 tsp.)
- Cumin (1 tsp.)
- Pepper (.25 tsp.)
- Salt (.25 tsp.)
- Eggs (10)
- Pepper Jack or your choice of cheese (1 cup)
- 1% milk (1 cup)

Ingredient List - Optional Toppings:
- Cilantro
- Salsa
- Sour cream
- Avocado

Prep Technique:
1. On the stovetop, use a skillet using the medium heat temperature setting to cook the sausage. Pour the salsa and seasonings into the skillet. When done, set aside to slightly cool.
2. Whisk the milk and eggs in another dish. Add the mixtures together and toss in the cheese. Mix well.
3. Coat the bottom of the cooker with a little cooking spray, and empty in the fixings.

4. Secure the lid and cook using the high setting for two and one-half hours or on low for five hours.
5. Add the desired toppings.

Oven-Baked Pancake With Bacon and Onions

Servings Provided: 4

Macro Counts Per Serving:
- **Calories**: 545
- **Protein**: 16 g
- **Fat Content**: 50 g
- **Total Net Carbs**: 5 g

Ingredient List:
- Turkey or pork bacon (3.5 oz.)
- Yellow onion (.5 of 1)
- Butter to fry in (2 tbsp.)
- Eggs (4)
- Heavy whipping cream (1 cup)
- Cottage cheese (.5 cup)
- Almond flour (.5 cup)
- Ground psyllium husk powder (1 tbsp.)
- Salt (1 tsp.)
- Baking powder (1 tsp.)
- *Optional*: Chopped fresh parsley - for garnish (1 tbsp.)

Prep Technique:
1. Warm up the oven to reach 350° Fahrenheit. Chop the onion and bacon.
2. Prepare a skillet and add the onion until they start crisping. Set aside.
3. Whisk the eggs, cream, and cottage cheese. Mix in with the baking powder, psyllium husk, salt, and almond flour. Let it rest for 2-3 minutes.
4. Pour the batter to the prepared pan and sprinkle with the crispy onion and bacon.
5. Bake until the center is set or about 20-25 minutes.

Quiche Cups

Servings Provided: 1 large

Macro Counts Per Serving:
- **Calories**: 105
- **Protein**: 12.8g
- **Fat Content**: 14.2 g
- **Total Net Carbs**: 2.1 g

Ingredient List:
- Frozen spinach (2 cups)
- Onion (.5 of 1)
- Egg Beaters (2 cups)
- Mozzarella cheese (.5 cup - shredded)
- Hot sauce (.5 tsp.)

Prep Technique:
1. Prepare a muffin tin with cooking spray or a paper liner.
2. Chop the spinach and slice the onion. Microwave both until the onion is soft, and the spinach is thawed.
3. Combine everything and sprinkle using the pepper and salt.
4. Bake at 375° Fahrenheit for 20 minutes.

Sausage Egg Muffin

Servings Provided: 1

Macro Counts Per Serving:

- **Calories**: 540
- **Protein**: 27 g
- **Fat Content**: 42 g
- **Total Net Carbs**: 3.5 g

Ingredient List:

- Heavy cream (1 tbsp.)
- Butter (melted (.5 tbsp.)
- Whisked egg (1 large)
- Ground flaxseed (2 tbsp.)
- Baking soda (.25 tsp.)
- Coconut flour (2 tsp.)
- Apple cider vinegar (.25 tsp.)
- Ground pork sausage (2 oz.)
- Egg (1 large)

Prep Technique:

1. Whisk together the heavy cream, butter, and egg in a greased 16-ounce ramekin.
2. Add the coconut flour, and ground flaxseed then whisk in the baking soda and cider vinegar.
3. Microwave on high heat for 1.5 minutes until firm. Turn out onto a plate.
4. Slice the bun in half and toast it in the toaster.
5. Shape the ground sausage into a patty the size of the bun and fry using the med-high heat setting until browned on both sides, turning as needed.
6. Place a round cookie cutter in another skillet and grease the inside with cooking spray.
7. Crack the egg into the cookie cutter and stir to break up the yolk. Cook using the med-high temperature setting until the egg is set.

8. Sandwich the sausage patty and cooked egg between the toasted bread slices and serve.

Single-Serve Baked Eggs

Servings Provided: 1

Macro Counts Per Serving:

- **Calories**: 174
- **Protein**: 10.7 g
- **Fat Content**: 14.3 g
- **Total Net Carbs**: 0.6 g

Ingredient List:

- Melted butter (1 tsp.)
- Bacon (1 slice)
- Egg (1)
- Keto-friendly cheese (.25 of 1 slice)

Prep Technique:

1. Set the oven temperature to 350° Fahrenheit.
2. Prepare the bacon using the med-hi heat setting on the stovetop. It should be browned but flexible.
3. Wrap a muffin cup with the prepared bacon. Drop in the butter, and then the egg.
4. Bake for 10 to 15 minutes. Serve.

Strawberry Donuts

Servings Provided: 12

Macro Counts Per Serving:
- **Calories**: 221
- **Protein**: 6 g
- **Fat Content**: 20.3 g
- **Total Net Carbs**: 0.6 g

Ingredient List - The Donuts:
- Blanched finely ground almond flour (2 cups)
- Unflavored protein powder (2 tbsp.)
- Baking powder (2 tsp.)
- Sugar-Free Strawberry Jell-O Powder (1 0.3 oz. packet)
- Butter (.5 cup)
- Cream cheese (2 oz.)
- Sour cream (.25 cup)
- Vanilla extract (1.5 tsp.)
- Erythritol (.5 cup)
- Strawberries (10)
- Lemon juice (2 tsp.)
- Water (2 tsp.)
- Egg whites (2)

Ingredient List -The Glaze:
- Strawberries (4)
- Heavy whipping cream (2 tbsp.)
- Powdered erythritol (2 tbsp.)
- Water (2 tsp.)

Prep Technique - The Donuts:
1. Heat oven to 350° Fahrenheit.
2. Butter or (or nonstick spray) your donut pan and set aside.
3. Whisk the almond flour, protein powder, baking powder, and sugar-free strawberry Jell-O powder in a mixing container. Set aside.

4. In a separate bowl, add butter and cream cheese. Microwave for 30 seconds to melt, being careful to not burn the cream cheese. Stir well.
5. Add sour cream, vanilla extract, and erythritol to the butter and cream cheese mixture. Stir well.
6. In a blender, puree strawberries, lemon juice, and water together until no lumps remain.
7. Combine all of the fixings and stir until very well combined.
8. Then, stir in the strawberry puree. Once combined, stir in egg whites until smooth.
9. Scoop batter into a freezer sized Ziploc bag. Twist the end of the bag to remove air then cut off a lower corner, and pipe the batter into a buttered donut pan. You will need 12 donut molds total, so either two 6-donut pans or work in batches.
10. Bake for 12 minutes. Cool completely before removing from donut pan. Otherwise, the donuts will crumble

Prep Technique - The Glaze:

1. Put the strawberries, heavy whipping cream and water into the blender then puree. Pour into a small bowl and whisk in erythritol.
2. Remove from blender and brush evenly across donuts. This glaze is more for extra flavor and moisture, so it's a little runny.

Chapter 4: Lunchtime Options

Salad Dishes

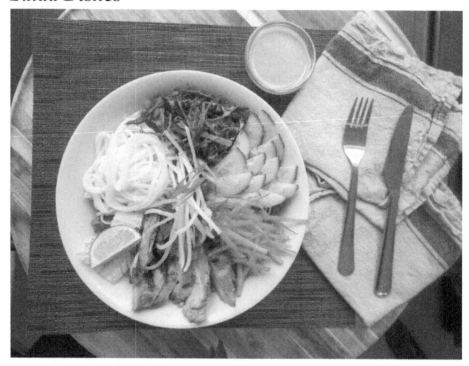

Asian Style Zucchini Salad

Servings Provided: 2

Macro Counts Per Serving:

- **Calories**: 846
- **Protein**: 14 g
- **Fat Content**: 86 g
- **Total Net Carbs**: 7 g

Ingredient List:

- Sesame oil (1.5 tbsp.)
- Almonds (.5 tbsp.)
- White vinegar (1 tbsp.)

- Crumbled feta cheese (.5 cup)
- Medium zucchini (1)
- Shredded cabbage (.5 cup)
- Sunflower seeds (1.5 tbsp.)

Prep Technique:
1. Roast the almonds in a deep-frying pan using the low-temperature setting.
2. Use a spiralizer to shred the zucchini into strips.
3. Prepare the salad using the cabbage, zucchini, almonds, and sunflower seeds.
4. Whisk both oils and the vinegar. Spritz over the salad.
5. Garnish with the feta and toss before serving.

Caprese Salad

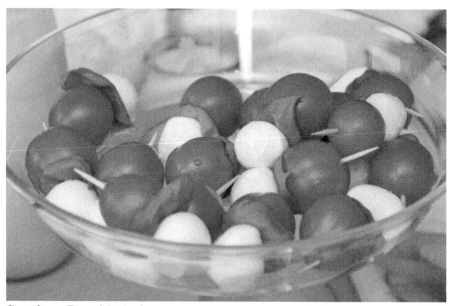

Servings Provided: 4

Macro Counts Per Serving:
- **Calories**: 190.75
- **Protein**: 7.7 g
- **Fat Content**: 63.5 g
- **Total Net Carbs**: 4.58 g

Ingredient List:
- Grape tomatoes (3 cups)
- Peeled garlic cloves (4)
- Avocado oil (2 tbsp.)
- Mozzarella balls (10 pearl-sized)
- Baby spinach leaves (4 cups)
- Brine reserved from the cheese (1 tbsp.)
- Fresh basil leaves (.25 cups)
- Pesto (1 tbsp.)

Prep Technique:

1. Use some aluminum foil to cover a baking tray. Program the oven to 400° Fahrenheit.
2. Arrange the cloves and tomatoes on the baking pan and drizzle with oil.
3. Bake until the tops are slightly browned (20-30 min.).
4. Drain the brine liquid (saving one tablespoon) from the mozzarella. Mix the pesto with the brine.
5. Arrange the spinach in a large serving bowl. Transfer the tomatoes to the dish along with the roasted garlic.
6. Drizzle with pesto sauce.
7. Garnish with the mozzarella balls, and freshly torn basil leaves.

Cauliflower and Shrimp Salad

Servings Provided: 6

Macro Counts Per Serving:
- **Calories**: 214
- **Protein**: 17 g
- **Fat Content**: 13 g
- **Total Net Carbs**: 5 g

Ingredient List:
- Medium raw shrimp (1 lb.)
- Cauliflower(1 head)
- Cucumbers (2)
- Fresh lemon juice (.25 cup)
- Olive oil (1 tbsp. + .25 cup)
- Freshly chopped dill (3 tbsp.)
- Grated lemon zest (2 tbsp.)

Prep Technique:
1. Peel, clean, and discard the tail from the shrimp. Arrange them on a baking tin, and sprinkle with 1 tbsp. of oil.
2. Roast at 350° Fahrenheit for approximately 8 to 10 minutes; remove when opaque.
3. Chop the cauliflower into small pieces and discard the head.
4. Microwave the florets in a shallow bowl for 5 minutes until they have a soft texture—not mushy. Let it cool.
5. Peel, remove the seeds and chop the cucumbers into ½-inch pieces.
6. After the shrimp have cooled; slice them lengthwise or chop them up.
7. Combine the cucumber, cauliflower, and the shrimp. Add the chopped dill and lemon zest.
8. *Note:* Hold the ¼ cup lemon juice or the remainder of the olive oil (1/4 cup) mixture that will be used as the dressing.

Chicken Salad With Kiwi and Feta

Servings Provided: 2

Macro Counts Per Serving:
- **Calories**: 314
- **Protein**: 28 g
- **Fat Content**: 15 g
- **Total Net Carbs**: 13 g

Ingredient List:
- Fig balsamic vinegar (1 tbsp.)
- Kiwis (2)
- Olive oil (1 tbsp.)
- Salt (1 pinch)
- Mixed field greens (4 cups)
- Chopped grilled chicken breast (1 cup - about 5 oz.)
- Feta cheese (.33 cup)

Prep Technique:
1. Chop the chicken and crumble the feta.
2. Whisk the balsamic vinegar, oil, and salt.
3. Add the greens and chicken breast.
4. Peel and cut the kiwi into halves. Dice into 1-inch wedges and add to the salad with the crumbled feta.
5. Toss well to combine.

Feta Cheese Salad With Balsamic Butter

Servings Provided:1

Macro Counts Per Serving:

- **Calories**: 609
- **Protein**: 16 g
- **Fat Content**: 70 g
- **Total Net Carbs**: 8 g

Ingredient List:

- Baby spinach (.5 cup)
- Crumbled feta cheese (.5 cup)
- Pumpkin seeds (.125 cup)
- Butter (.25 cup)
- Balsamic vinegar (1 tbsp.)

Prep Technique:

1. Warm the oven to reach 400° Fahrenheit.
2. Lightly spritz the baking tray with cooking oil spray.
3. Crumble the cheese onto the pan. Bake for about 10 minutes.
4. Use the high-temperature setting on the stovetop to heat a dry skillet. Toast the seeds until they begin to pop.
5. Reduce the temperature and add the butter. Simmer until golden brown and add the vinegar. Simmer for about two minutes and turn off the burner.
6. Arrange the baby spinach leaves on a salad dish.
7. Pour butter over that and top with feta cheese before serving.

Loaded Cauliflower Bowl

Servings Provided: 4

Macro Counts Per Serving:
- **Calories**: 329
- **Protein**: 18 g
- **Fat Content**: 27 g
- **Total Net Carbs**: 3 g

Ingredient List:
- Fresh cauliflower (2 cups)
- Butter (3 tbsp.)
- Pickled jalapeno slices (.25 cup)
- Diced onion (.25 cup)
- Cooked brisket (2 cups)
- Shredded sharp cheddar (1 cup)
- Cream cheese - softened (2 oz.)
- Heavy cream (.25 cup)
- Crumbled bacon (.25 cup)
- Sliced green onions (2 tbsp.)

Prep Technique:
1. Slice or dice the cauliflower into small pieces. Prepare using your favorite method until fork-tender. Set aside.
2. In a skillet, set the temperature setting to medium to melt the butter. Toss in the onion, and jalapeno slices. Sauté until the onions are translucent.
3. Lower the heat slightly and add the cooked brisket and cream cheese. Stir until the cheese is melted.
4. Turn off the heat. Add heavy cream, cauliflower, and sharp cheddar.
5. Stir until well mixed.
6. Sprinkle with green onions and crumbled bacon. Serve.

Loaded Chicken Salad

Servings Provided: 4

Macro Counts Per Serving:
- **Calories**: 430
- **Protein**: 31.73 g
- **Fat Content**: 29.36 g
- **Total Net Carbs**: 6.74 g

Ingredient List:
- Avocado (1)
- Large tomato (1 any color)
- Artichoke hearts (6 oz.)
- Red onion (.5 of 1)
- Asparagus (5)
- Basil (20 leaves)
- Baby spinach (4 cups)
- Mozzarella balls (3.5 oz.)
- Chicken breast (1 - about 11 oz. - boneless - with or without skin)
- Olive oil (1 tbsp.)
- Black pepper and Himalayan salt (.25 tsp.)

Ingredient List - The Dressing

- Clove garlic (1)
- Himalayan salt (1 pinch)
- Black pepper (as desired)
- Dijon mustard (1 tsp.)
- Olive oil (2 tbsp.)
- Balsamic vinegar (1.5 tbsp.)

Prep Technique:
1. Prepare the veggies. Slice the red onion. Use a sharp knife to remove the skin from the avocado and dice. Dice the tomato and mince the garlic. Roll and slice the basil leaves. Cut the stems from the asparagus and slice into halves.

2. Slice the chicken breast in half lengthwise with a dusting of salt and pepper.
3. Pour one tablespoon of olive oil into a cast-iron skillet. When it's hot, arrange the prepared chicken in the pan and fry for three minutes per side.
4. Add the asparagus and cook a few minutes until softened. Transfer and cool to slice.
5. Combine the olive oil, balsamic vinegar, mustard, salt, pepper, and minced garlic.
6. Arrange the baby spinach onto a large platter. Cover with the grilled chicken, avocado, red onions, tomatoes, artichoke, asparagus, mozzarella, and basil.
7. Serve with a portion of dressing.

Salad Sandwiches

Servings Provided: 1

Macro Counts Per Serving:
- **Calories**: 374
- **Protein**: 10 g
- **Fat Content**: 34 g
- **Total Net Carbs**: 3 g

Ingredient List:
- Romaine lettuce (2 oz.)
- Butter (.5 oz.)
- Edam or your favorite cheese (1 oz.)
- Cherry tomato (1)
- Avocado (.5 of 1)

Prep Technique:
1. Rinse the lettuce, and arrange in a colander to drain.
2. Toss the lettuce into a salad dish and smear with the butter, cheese, avocado slices, and tomato on top.
3. Serve any time for a delicious meal or snack.

Shrimp Avocado Salad With Tomatoes and Feta

Servings Provided: 2

Macro Counts Per Serving:
- **Calories**: 430
- **Protein**: 24 g
- **Fat Content**: 33 g
- **Total Net Carbs**: 6.5 g

Ingredient List:
- Shrimp (8 oz.)
- Large avocado (1 diced)
- Beefsteak tomato (1 small)
- Feta cheese (.33 cup)
- Olive oil (1 tbsp.)
- Cilantro/parsley (.33 cup)
- Salted butter (2 tbsp. - melted)
- Black pepper and salt (.25 tsp. each)
- Lemon juice (1 tbsp.)

Prep Technique:
1. Devein the shrimp, peel, and pat dry. Dice and drain the tomato, chop the parsley, and crumble the feta.
2. Melt the butter and toss the shrimp in a bowl until well-coated.
3. Warm a pan using the med-high heat setting until hot.
4. Toss the shrimp into the pan in a single layer, searing until it starts to become pink around the edges (1 min.). Flip and cook until the shrimp are cooked through (30 sec. approx.).
5. Transfer the shrimp to a plate to cool.
6. Add all other fixings into a large mixing bowl (diced tomato, diced avocado, olive oil, feta cheese, lemon juice, cilantro, salt, and pepper. Toss to mix.
7. Toss the shrimp and stir to mix together to serve.

Steak Salad

Servings Provided: 2

Macro Counts Per Serving:
- **Calories**: 403
- **Protein**: 25 g
- **Fat Content**: 33 g
- **Total Net Carbs**: 1.5 g

Ingredient List:
- Ribeye steak (1- 8 oz.)
- Green salad mix (2 cups)
- Olive oil (1 tbsp.)
- Steakhouse seasoning (1 tbsp.)
- Wine vinegar (1 tsp.)
- Pepper and salt (to taste)

Prep Technique:
1. Use the steak seasoning to prepare the steak and cook to your liking. Let it rest until cooled.
2. Arrange all of the salad fixings and sprinkle with pepper and salt.
3. Toss and drizzle with oil.
4. Slice the steak into bite-sized strips.
5. Place the salad on two serving dishes and sprinkle the steak bits on top.
6. Use your favorite dressing if desired - but count the carbs.

Swedish Dill Shrimp Salad

Servings Provided: 4

Macro Counts Per Serving:
- **Calories**: 496
- **Protein**: 14 g
- **Fat Content**: 48 g
- **Total Net Carbs**: 2 g

Ingredient List:
- Shrimp, peeled and cooked (10 oz.)
- Mayonnaise (1 cup)
- Sour cream or crème Fraiche (.25 cup)
- Fresh dill (2 tbsp.)
- Fish roe (2 oz.)
- Lemon juice (2 tsp.)
- Black pepper and salt (to your liking)

Prep Technique:
1. Roughly chop half of the shrimp.
2. Combine the sour cream and mayonnaise in a mixing container.
3. Fold in the dill, roe, and shrimp. Reserve a portion for garnishing.
4. Sprinkle using pepper and salt.
5. Drizzle with lemon juice before serving.

Soup and Chili

Asiago Tomato Soup

Servings Provided: 4
Macro Counts Per Serving:
- **Calories**: 302
- **Protein**: 9 g
- **Fat Content**: 26 g
- **Total Net Carbs**: 8.75 g

Ingredient List:
- Tomato paste (1 small can)
- Garlic (1 tsp.)
- Oregano (1 tsp.)
- Heavy whipping cream (1 cup)
- Water (.25 cup)
- Pepper and salt (as desired)
- Asiago cheese (.75 cup)

Prep Technique:
1. Mince the garlic and combine with the tomato paste in a Dutch oven and add the cream. Gently whisk.
2. As it begins to boil, blend in small amounts of cheese. Pour in the water and simmer 4 to 5 minutes.
3. Stir well and serve.

Broccoli Cheddar Soup

Servings Provided: 4

Macro Counts Per Serving:
- **Calories**: 285
- **Protein**: 12 g
- **Fat Content**: 24 g
- **Total Net Carbs**: 2 g

Ingredient List:
- Butter (2 tbsp.)
- White onion (.125 tsp.)
- Garlic - finely minced (.5 tsp.)
- Chicken broth (2 cups)
- Salt and Pepper (to your liking)
- Broccoli - chopped into bite-size pieces (1 cup)
- Cream cheese (1 tbsp.)
- Heavy whipping cream (.25 cup)
- Cheddar cheese (1 cup - shredded)
- *Optional*: Bacon - Cooked and Crumbled (2 slices)
- *Optional:* Xanthan gum - for thickening (.5 tsp.)

Prep Technique:
1. Prepare a skillet using the medium heat temperature setting. Add the butter.
2. Toss in the garlic and onion to sauté until the onions become translucent.
3. Pour in the broccoli and broth. Simmer with the pepper, salt, and seasonings of choice.
4. Add the cream cheese in a microwave-safe bowl. Microwave until softened and easily stirred (30 sec.).
5. Stir heavy whipping cream and cream cheese into the soup; bring to a boil.
6. Turn off the heat. Stir in cheddar cheese and xanthan gum for thickening.
7. Serve hot with bacon crumbles.

Egg Drop Soup

Servings Provided: 6

Macro Counts Per Serving:
- **Calories**: 255
- **Protein**: 11 g
- **Fat Content**: 22 g
- **Total Net Carbs**: 3 g

Ingredient List:
- Vegetable broth (2 quarts)
- Freshly chopped ginger (1 tbsp.)
- Turmeric (1 tbsp.)
- Sliced chili pepper (1 small)
- Coconut aminos (2 tbsp.)
- Minced garlic cloves (2)
- Large eggs (4)
- Mushrooms (2 cups sliced)
- Chopped spinach (4 cups)
- Sliced spring onions (2 medium)
- Freshly chopped cilantro (2 tbsp.)
- Black pepper (to your liking)
- Pink Himalayan (1 tsp.)
- *For Serving:* Olive oil (6 tbsp.)

Prep Technique:
1. Grate the ginger root and turmeric. Mince the garlic cloves and slice the peppers and mushrooms.
2. Chop the chard stalks and leaves. Separate the stalks from the leaves.
3. Dump the vegetable stock into a soup pot and simmer until it begins to boil. Toss in the garlic, ginger, turmeric, chard stalks, mushrooms, coconut aminos, and chili peppers. Boil for approximately five minutes.
4. Fold in the chard leaves and simmer for one minute.
5. Whip the eggs in a dish and add them slowly to the soup mixture. Stir until the egg is done and set it on the

countertop.

6. Slice the onions and chop the cilantro. Toss them into the pot.
7. Pour into serving bowls and drizzle with some olive oil (1 tbsp. per serving).
8. Serve warm or chilled.

No Beans Beef Chili

Servings Provided: 6

Macro Counts Per Serving:
- **Calories**: 263
- **Protein**: 26 g
- **Fat Content**: 14 g
- **Total Net Carbs**: 5 g

Ingredient List:
- Water (3 cups)
- Ground beef 1.5 lb.)
- Bay leaves (3)
- Chili powder (2 tbsp.)
- Salt (1.5 tsp.)
- Allspice (.5 tsp.)
- Red pepper (.5 tsp.)
- Tomato paste (6 oz.)
- Sliced black olives (2.25 oz.)
- Finely chopped chili peppers (.25 cup)
- Cumin (.75 tsp.)
- Black pepper (.75 tsp.)
- Cinnamon (.25 tsp.)
- Minced garlic cloves (2)
- Chopped onion (.25 cup)
- Worcestershire sauce (1 tsp.)

Prep Technique:
1. Break apart the ground beef in a large stew pot on the stovetop. Drain away the juices.
2. Combine with the rest of the fixings. Bring to a boil.
3. Simmer two hours and serve.

Vietnamese Shirataki Soup

Servings Provided: 2

Macro Counts Per Serving:
- **Calories**: 130
- **Protein**: 1 g
- **Fat Content**: 12 g
- **Total Net Carbs**: 1.5 g

Ingredient List:
- Boneless - skinless chicken thighs (2)
- Chicken stock (3 cups)
- Minced ginger (1 tsp.)
- Cardamom (.25 tsp.)
- Minced garlic clove (1)
- Mushrooms – your choice (.5 cup)
- *Optional*: Chili sauce (1 tsp.)
- Chopped cilantro (to taste)
- Thinly sliced chili pepper (1)

Prep Technique:
1. On the stovetop, use the med-high heat setting to warm up the stock.
2. Toss in the ginger, garlic, mushrooms, and cardamom. Simmer for about ten minutes.
3. Fold in the chicken. Cook for about five minutes or until done.
4. Prepare two soup dishes and add the sliced chili pepper to each dish. Serve the soup and garnish with the cilantro.
5. Adjust the spices to your liking.

White Chicken Chili

Servings Provided: 4

Macro Counts Per Serving:
- **Calories**: 481
- **Protein**: 39 g
- **Fat Content**: 30 g
- **Total Net Carbs**: 4 g

Ingredient List:
- Chicken breast (1 lb.)
- Chicken broth (1.5 cups)
- Garlic cloves (2)
- Green chiles (4.5 oz. can)
- Jalapeno (1)
- Green pepper (1)
- Onion (.25 cup)
- Butter (4 tbsp.)
- Heavy whipping cream (.25 cup)
- Cream cheese (4 oz.)
- Cumin (2 tsp.)
- Oregano (1 tsp.)
- *Optional*: Cayenne (.25 tsp.)
- Black pepper and salt (as desired)

Prep Technique:
1. Dice the onion, chiles, jalapeno, and green pepper. Mince the garlic.
2. Season the chicken with pepper, salt, cayenne, oregano, and cumin. Add it to a large skillet.
3. Sear both sides using the medium heat temperature setting until golden.
4. Pour the broth into the pot, cover. Simmer the chicken fixings for 15-20 minutes until done.
5. Meanwhile, melt butter in a skillet.
6. Dice and add the green pepper, jalapeno, chiles, and onion into the skillet. Sauté until the veggies are softened.

7. Mince and add the garlic. Sauté an additional 30 seconds and extinguish the heat. Set aside.
8. Once the chicken is done, shred and add back into the broth.
9. Add the sautéed veggies and simmer for about 10 minutes.
10. Soften the cream cheese in a microwave until you can stir it (20 sec.).
11. Mix the cream cheese with the heavy whipping cream.
12. Add the mixture into the pot with the chicken and veggies.
13. Simmer for another 15 minutes.
14. Serve with your favorite toppings such as avocado slices, cilantro, or sour cream.

Other Luncheon Favorites

Bacon and Shrimp Risotto

Servings Provided: 2
Macro Counts Per Serving:
- **Calories**: 224
- **Protein**: 23.7 g
- **Fat Content**: 9.4 g
- **Total Net Carbs**: 5.3 g

Ingredient List:
- Chopped bacon (4 slices)
- Daikon/winter radish/ jicama (2 cups)
- Dry white wine (2 tbsp.)
- Chicken stock (.25 cup)
- Garlic clove (1)
- Ground pepper (as desired)
- Chopped parsley (2 tbsp.)
- Cooked shrimp (4 oz.)

Prep Technique:
1. Cut the skin of the radish and slice. Mince the garlic, and chop the bacon. Remove as much water as possible from the daikon once it's shredded.
2. On the stovetop, warm up a saucepan using the medium heat setting. Toss in the bacon and fry until it's crispy. Leave the drippings in the pan and remove the bacon to drain.
3. Add the wine, daikon, salt, pepper, stock, and garlic into the pan and cook six to eight minutes until most of the liquid is absorbed.
4. Fold in the bacon (save a few bits for the topping), and shrimp along with the parsley.
5. Serve and enjoy.

6. *Note*: If you cannot find the daikon, you can also substitute using some shredded cauliflower in its place.

Beef and Cheddar Platter

Servings Provided: 2

Macro Counts Per Serving:
- **Calories**: 1072
- **Protein**: 38 g
- **Fat Content**: 98 g
- **Total Net Carbs**: 6 g

Ingredient List:
- Deli roast beef (7 oz.)
- Cheddar cheese (5 oz.)
- Avocado (1)
- Radishes (6)
- Scallion (1)
- Mayonnaise (.5 cup)
- Dijon mustard (1 tbsp.)
- Lettuce (2 oz.)
- Olive oil (2 tbsp.)
- Salt and pepper (to your liking)

Prep Technique:
1. Slice the onion.
2. Place the cheese, roast beef, radishes, and avocado on a serving platter.
3. Add the sliced onion, a dollop of mayo, and mustard.
4. Serve with lettuce and a spritz of olive oil.

Black Bean Quiche

Servings Provided: 6

Macro Counts Per Serving:
- **Calories**: 141.7
- **Protein**:10 g
- **Fat Content**: 8.7 g
- **Total Net Carbs**: 5.1 g

Ingredient List:
- Eggs (5 whole and 5 whites)
- Salt (.5 tsp.)
- Water (.33 cup)
- Black pepper (.25 tsp.)
- Chopped tomato (.5 cup)
- Low-sodium black beans (.66 cup)
- Grated jack cheese (3 oz.)
- *For the Garnish*: Cilantro

Prep Technique:
1. Whisk all of the eggs with the salt, pepper, and water.
2. Warm up the oven to 375° Fahrenheit.
3. Empty the mixture into a greased pie dish coated with a spritz of cooking oil spray.
4. Sprinkle with the beans, tomatoes, and cheese.
5. Bake for 30 to 35 minutes until the centers of the eggs are set.
6. Let them cool for about ten minutes and sprinkle using the cilantro before serving.

Broccoli and Tuna

Servings Provided: 2

Macro Counts Per Serving:
- **Calories**: 122
- **Protein**: 14.2 g
- **Fat Content**: 20.6 g
- **Total Net Carbs**: 3 g

Ingredient List:
- Light tuna (3 oz. can)
- Broccoli (1 cup)
- Cheese (2 tbsp.)
- Salt (1 tsp.)

Prep Technique:
1. Place the frozen florets of broccoli into a pan of water until they're thawed. Drain.
2. Mix the broccoli and cheese until melted. Fold in the tuna.
3. Salt if desired.
4. Serve any time for a great treat.

Cauliflower and Mushroom Risotto

Servings Provided: 4

Macro Counts Per Serving:
- **Calories**: 186
- **Protein**: 1 g
- **Fat Content**: 17.1 g
- **Total Net Carbs**: 4.3 g

Ingredient List:
- Grated head of cauliflower (1)
- Vegetable stock (1 cup)
- Chopped mushrooms (9 oz.)
- Butter (2 tbsp.)
- Coconut cream (1 cup)
- Pepper and Salt (to taste)

Prep Technique:
1. Pour the stock in a saucepan. Boil and set aside.
2. Prepare a skillet with butter. Sauté the mushrooms until golden.
3. Grate and stir in the cauliflower and stock.
4. Simmer and add the cream, cooking until the cauliflower is al dente. Serve.

Chicken Sausage Corn Dogs

Servings Provided: 4

Macro Counts Per Serving:
- **Calories**: 494
- **Protein**:15.4 g
- **Fat Content**: 45.9 g
- **Total Net Carbs**: 4.5 g

Ingredient List:
- Chicken sausage (4 links)
- Lard (1.5 cups)
- Almond flour (1 cup)
- Ms. Dash Table Blend (1 tsp.)
- Kosher salt (.5 tsp.)
- Baking powder (1 tsp.)
- Turmeric (.5 tsp.)
- Cayenne pepper (.25 tsp.)
- Large eggs (2)
- Heavy whipping cream (2 tbsp.)
- *For the Pan*: Oil (1.5 cups)

Prep Technique:
1. Combine the spices and almond meal.
2. In another dish, whisk the heavy cream, egg, and add the baking powder to the mixture.
3. Heat a saucepan with the oil (400° Fahrenheit approximately).
4. Dip the dogs/sausages into the mixture and add them to the oil. Fry for approximately two minutes for each side.
5. Transfer to a plate of paper towels to drain. Serve.

Grilled Buffalo Chicken Lettuce Wraps

Servings Provided: 15

Macro Counts Per Serving:
- **Calories**: 53
- **Protein**: 5 g
- **Fat Content**: 3 g
- **Total Net Carbs**: 2 g

Ingredient List:
- Franks Red Hot Sauce (.75 cup)
- Boneless and skinless breasts of chicken (3 large)
- Lettuce cups (15)
- Avocado (1 diced)
- Cherry tomatoes (.75 cup)
- Ranch dressing (.5 cup)
- Sliced green onions (.25 cup)
- *Also Needed*: Grill basket or kabob sticks

Prep Technique:
1. Dice up the chicken into ½- inch cubes. Slice the tomatoes into halves. Set aside for now.
2. Place the chicken in a dish and add Frank's sauce (or your choice). Put a lid or foil over the container and put it in the refrigerator for about 30 minutes.
3. Set the grill temperature to 400° Fahrenheit.
4. Arrange the grill basket with the chicken/kabobs on the grill and cook for 8-10 minutes. Stir constantly. Take them from the grill and dump them into a container with the remainder of the buffalo sauce.
5. Prepare the lettuce cups with two to three cubes of chicken, two to three diced tomatoes, a pinch of onions, two to three diced avocados, and a drizzle of dressing.

Halloumi Burger

Servings Provided: 4

Macro Counts Per Serving:
- **Calories**: 534
- **Protein**: 23.8 g
- **Fat Content**: 45.1 g
- **Total Net Carbs**: 9.4 g

Ingredient List:
- Sour cream (6.7 tbsp.)
- Mayonnaise (6.7 tbsp.)
- Coconut oil or butter for the pan
- Halloumi cheese (15 oz.)
- Sliced veggies (your choice)

Prep Technique:
1. Whisk the mayo and sour cream and cover the bowl. Store in the fridge.
2. Add the butter to a skillet and add cheese. Cook until lightly browned.
3. Place on a plate and garnish with the mayo mix and veggies. Serve.

Lemon Garlic Shrimp Pasta

Servings Provided: 4

Macro Counts Per Serving:
- **Calories**: 360
- **Protein**: 36 g
- **Fat Content**: 21 g
- **Total Net Carbs**: 3.5 g

Ingredient List:
- Angel hair pasta (2 bags)
- Garlic cloves (4)
- Olive oil (2 tbsp.)
- Butter (2 tbsp.)
- Lemon (.5 of 1)
- Large raw shrimp (1 lb.)
- Paprika (.5 tsp.)
- Fresh basil (as desired)
- Pepper and salt (as desired)

Prep Technique:
1. Drain the water from the package of noodles and rinse them in cold water. Add them to a pot of boiling water for two minutes. Transfer to a hot skillet over medium heat to remove the excess liquid (dry roast). Set them aside.
2. Use the same pan to warm the butter, oil, and mashed garlic. Sauté for a few minutes, but *don't* brown.
3. Slice the lemon into rounds and add them to the garlic along with the shrimp. Sauté for approximately three minutes per side.
4. Add the noodles and spices and stir to blend the flavors.

Chapter 5: Dinner Specialties

Chicken and Poultry Favorites

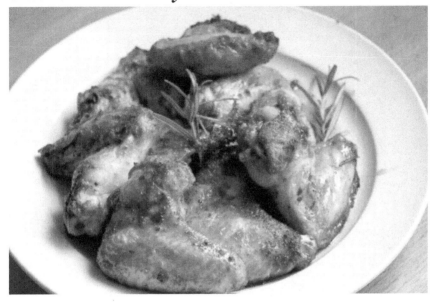

Baked Whole Turkey

Servings Provided: 10

Macro Counts Per Serving:
- **Calories**: 391
- **Protein**: 42 g
- **Fat Content**: 23g
- **Total Net Carbs**: 1 g

Ingredient List:
- Olive oil (4 tbsp.)
- Turkey (10 lb.)
- Garlic powder (2 tsp.)
- Salt (2 tsp.)
- Thyme (1 tsp.)
- Paprika (1 tsp.)
- Pepper (1 tsp.)
- Reduced-sodium chicken broth (.5 cup)

Prep Technique:
1. Rinse and pat dry the turkey, removing the giblets.
2. Grease a roasting pan and set the oven temperature to 325° Fahrenheit.
3. Cover the turkey with a rub of the seasonings and oil.
4. Arrange the turkey in the pan along with the broth.
5. Bake for three hours (internal temperature – 165° Fahrenheit.). Baste every hour or so to prevent dryness.
6. Let the turkey stand about 30 minutes before slicing to serve.
7. Add a little rosemary, or add a bit more thyme for a taste change.

Balsamic Chicken Thighs - Slow Cooked

Servings Provided: 8

Macro Counts Per Serving:
- **Calories**: 133
- **Protein**: 20.1 g
- **Fat Content**: 4 g
- **Total Net Carbs**: 3.6 g

Ingredient List:
- Boneless chicken thighs (8 - 24 oz. approx.)
- Minced cloves of garlic (4)
- Dried minced onion (2 tsp.)
- Olive oil (1 tbsp.)
- Garlic powder (1 tsp.)
- Dried basil (1 tsp.)
- Pepper and Salt (.5 tsp. each)
- Balsamic vinegar (.5 cup)
- Sprinkle of freshly chopped parsley

Prep Technique:
1. Mix all of the dry spices (minced onion, pepper, salt, basil, and garlic powder). Rub over the chicken and set aside for now.
2. Pour the extra-virgin olive oil and garlic into the slow cooker and add the chicken.
3. Empty the vinegar over the thighs and place the lid securely closed.
4. Cook for four hours using the high-temperature setting.
5. Sprinkle using the freshly chopped parsley, serve, and enjoy.

Chicken Enchilada Bowl

Servings Provided: 4

Macro Counts Per Serving:
- **Calories**: 568
- **Protein**: 38.38g
- **Fat Content**: 40.21g
- **Total Net Carbs**: 6.14 g

Ingredient List:
- Coconut oil - for searing chicken (2 tbsp.)
- Boneless - skinless chicken thighs (1 lb.)
- Red enchilada sauce (.75 cup)
- Water (.25 cup)
- Chopped onion (.25 cup)
- Diced green chiles (4 oz. can)

Ingredient List - Toppings:

- Avocado (1 whole - diced)
- Shredded mild cheddar cheese (1 cup)
- Chopped pickled jalapenos (.25 cup)
- Sour cream (.5 cup)
- Roma tomato (1 chopped)

Optional: Serve over plain cauliflower rice (or *Mexican cauliflower rice*) for a more complete meal!

Prep Technique:
1. Melt the coconut oil using the medium heat setting in a Dutch oven or stew pot. Add the thighs. Sear until lightly browned and add the water, enchilada sauce, chiles, and onions.
2. Lower the heat and simmer for 17-25 minutes until the center reaches 165° Fahrenheit internally.
3. Remove the chicken and chop. Add it back into the pot to simmer for about ten additional minutes.

4. Top with avocado, cheese, jalapeno, sour cream, tomato, and any other desired toppings. Serve alone or over cauliflower rice if desired.

Grilled Chicken With Spinach and Mozzarella

Servings Provided: 6

Macro Counts Per Serving:

- **Calories**: 195
- **Protein**: 30.9 g
- **Fat Content**: 6.1 g
- **Total Net Carbs**: 3.7 g

Ingredient List:

- Large chicken breasts (24 oz. or 6 portions)
- Olive oil (1 tsp.)
- Pepper and Kosher salt (as desired)
- Garlic cloves (3 crushed)
- Drained frozen spinach (10 oz.)
- Roasted red pepper strips packed in water (.5 cup)
- Shredded part-skim mozzarella (3 oz.)
- Olive oil cooking spray

Prep Technique:

1. Warm the oven to 400° Fahrenheit.
2. Prepare the grill/grill pan with the oil.
3. Sprinkle the salt and pepper onto the chicken. Cook about two to three minutes per side.
4. Add the oil into a frying pan along with the garlic. Continue cooking for about 30 seconds, add a sprinkle of salt and pepper, and toss in the spinach. Sauté another two to three minutes.
5. Arrange the chicken on a baking sheet and add the spinach to each one. Top them off with half of the cheese and peppers. Bake for about three minutes until lightly toasted.
6. Serve.

Herbal Green Beans and Chicken

Servings Provided: 3

Macro Counts Per Serving:

- **Calories**: 196
- **Protein**: 19 g
- **Fat Content**: 11 g
- **Total Net Carbs**: 4 g

Ingredient List:

- Olive oil (2 tbsp.)
- Trimmed green beans (1 cup)
- Whole chicken breasts (2)
- Cherry tomatoes (8 halve)
- Italian seasoning (1 tbsp.)
- Salt and pepper (1 tsp. of each)

Prep Technique:

1. Warm a skillet using the medium heat setting; add the oil.
2. Sprinkle the chicken with the pepper, Italian seasoning, and salt.
3. Arrange in the skillet for 10 minutes per side – or until thoroughly done.
4. Add the tomatoes and beans. Simmer another 5 to 7 minutes and serve.

Instant Pot Chicken Adobo

Servings Provided: 4

Macro Counts Per Serving:
- **Calories**: 370
- **Protein**: 37 g
- **Fat Content**: 21 g
- **Total Net Carbs**: 6.5g

Ingredient List:
- Chicken thighs (2 - 2.5 lb.)
- Low-sodium soy sauce (.5 cup)
- White vinegar (.33 cup)
- Sliced onion (1)
- Garlic (5 minced cloves)
- Bay leaves (3)
- Olive oil (2 tbsp.)
- Cayenne (.25 tsp.)
- Salt and coarse black pepper (to your liking)

Ingredient List - For Serving - Optional:

- Scallions (2 sliced)
- Cooked cauliflower rice

Prep Technique:
1. Select the sauté function on the Instant Pot.
2. Remove the skin and bones from the chicken. Generously season chicken thighs using the pepper and salt.
3. Pour the oil into the pot.
4. Arrange half of the chicken thighs in the pot and sauté for a couple of minutes per side Place on a platter and continue the process until done.
5. Pour in the vinegar, soy sauce, garlic, onion, and cayenne. Stir well and scrape any browned bits in the pot.
6. Add the chicken in a single layer, placing them on top of the onions, and toss in the bay leaves. Securely close the lid.

7. Cook for 10 minutes using the high-pressure function. Quick-release the steam and switch to the sauté function. Toss the bay leaves.
8. Sauté for another 15 minutes to thicken the sauce.
9. Serve the chicken and sauce, with cooked cauliflower rice and scallions.

Pan-Glazed Chicken and Basil

Servings Provided: 4

Macro Counts Per Serving:
- **Calories**: 161
- **Protein**: 26.2 g
- **Fat Content**: 4.7 g
- **Total Net Carbs**: 4.6 g

Ingredient List:
- Chicken breast halves (4- 4-oz.)
- Balsamic vinegar (2 tbsp.)
- Olive oil (2 tsp.)
- Dried Basil (2 tsp.)
- Black pepper and salt (.25 tsp. each)
- Honey (1 tbsp.)

Prep Technique:
1. Spice up the chicken with sea salt for a coarser salt. You can also add pepper.
2. Place the chicken in a large pan with oil using a med-high burner for about 4 or 5 minutes on each side.
3. Flip the chicken, and simmer for an extra five minutes or so. Mix and pour the vinegar, basil, and honey over the chicken. Continue cooking for 1 minute.

Slow-Cooked Teriyaki

Servings Provided: 6

Macro Counts Per Serving:
- **Calories**: 158
- **Protein**: 20 g
- **Fat Content**: 6 g
- **Total Net Carbs**: 4 g

Ingredient List:
- Chicken thighs (2 lb.)
- Red pepper (2)
- Yellow onion (1)
- Garlic cloves (3)
- Reduced-sodium beef broth (.5 cup)
- Coconut aminos (.25 cup)
- Water (.33 cup)
- Knob freshly grated ginger (1-inch piece)
- Pepper and salt (as desired)
- *For the Garnish*: 4 green onions
- *Optional for Serving*: Lettuce leaves

Prep Technique:
1. Chop the peppers, onions, and garlic.
2. Whisk the water, aminos, and broth – adding it to the cooker.
3. Blend in the rest of the fixings (omit the lettuce and green onions).
4. Cook for six hours using the high heat setting.
5. When done; garnish with onions, as is, or, on a bed of lettuce to create a delicious taco.

Thai Green Chicken Curry – Instant Pot

Servings Provided: 6

Macro Counts Per Serving:
- **Calories**: 231
- **Protein**: 17 g
- **Fat Content**: 15 g
- **Total Net Carbs**: 5 g

Ingredient List:
- Chicken thighs – remove skin and bones (1 lb.)
- Curry paste (2 tbsp.)
- Coconut oil (1 tbsp.)
- Minced garlic (1 tbsp.)
- Minced ginger (1 tbsp.)
- Sliced onion (.5 cup)
- Basil leaves (.5 cup)
- Peeled – chopped eggplant (2 cups)
- Chopped yellow, green or orange pepper (1)
- Unsweetened coconut milk (1 cup)
- Splenda/another sweetener (2 tbsp.)
- Soy sauce/coconut aminos (2 tbsp.)
- Salt (1 tbsp.)
- Fish sauce (1 tbsp.)

Prep Technique:
1. Set the Instant Pot on the sauté function. When hot, add the oil, and curry paste. Sauté for one to two minutes.
2. Toss in the garlic and ginger. Sauté for about 30 seconds. Stir in the onions along with the rest of the fixings. Deglaze the pan.
3. Switch to the slow cooker mode for 8 hours using the medium setting.
4. Stir and enjoy!

Beef Options

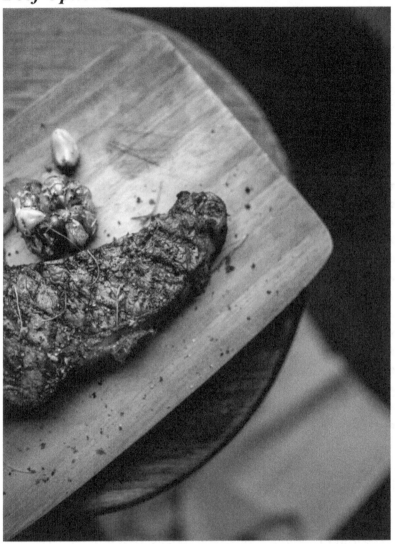

Bacon Burger and Cabbage Stir Fry

Servings Provided: 10

Macro Counts Per Serving:
- **Calories**: 357
- **Protein**:31.9 g
- **Fat Content**: 21.9 g
- **Total Net Carbs**: 4.5 g

Ingredient List:
- Ground beef (1 lb.)
- Bacon (1 lb.)
- Small onion (1)
- Cloves of garlic (3)
- Small head of cabbage (1 lb.)
- Black pepper (.25 tsp.)
- Sea salt (.5 tsp.)

Prep Technique:
1. Chop the bacon and onion. Mince the garlic.
2. Combine the beef and bacon in a wok or large skillet. Prepare until done and store in a bowl to keep warm.
3. Toss the minced garlic and onion into the hot grease. Add the cabbage and stir-fry until wilted. Blend in the meat and combine. Sprinkle with the pepper and salt as desired. Serve.

Barbacoa Beef

Servings Provided: 9

Macro Counts Per Serving:
- **Calories**: 153
- **Protein**: 24 g
- **Fat Content**: 4.5 g
- **Total Net Carbs**: 2 g

Ingredient List:
- Med. onion (.5 of 1)
- Garlic (5 cloves)
- Chipotles in adobo sauce (2-4)
- Lime (1 juiced)
- Cumin (1 tbsp.)
- Oregano (1 tbsp.)
- Water (1 cup)
- Ground cloves (.5 tsp.)
- Bay leaves (3)
- Kosher salt (2.5 tsp.)
- Black pepper (as desired)
- Eye of round/bottom round (3 lb.)
- Oil (1 tsp.)

Prep Technique:
1. In a blender, puree the onion, garlic cloves, lime juice, water, cloves, chipotles, cumin, and oregano – until smooth.
2. Remove all fat from the meat and chop into 3-inch bits. Season with 2 teaspoons of salt and a pinch of pepper.
3. Prepare an Instant Pot using the sauté setting and add the oil. Brown the meat in batches (5 min.). Add the sauce from the blender, and the bay leaves into the Instant Pot.
4. Secure the lid and set the timer for 65 minutes using the high-pressure setting. Natural or quick release the pressure and shred the beef with two forks. Reserve the juices and throw the bay leaves in the trash.

5. Return the meat to the pot with the cumin, salt to taste, and 1.5 cups of the reserved juices. Serve when hot.

Beef and Broccoli - Slow Cooked

Servings Provided: 4

Macro Counts Per Serving:
- **Calories**: 430
- **Protein**: 54 g
- **Fat Content**: 19 g
- **Total Net Carbs**: 3 g

Ingredient List:
- Liquid aminos (.66 cup)
- Flank steak (2 lb.)
- Beef broth (1 cup)
- Freshly grated ginger (1 tsp.)
- Keto-friendly sweetener - your choice (3 tbsp.)
- Minced garlic (3 cloves)
- Salt (.5 tsp.)
- Red pepper flakes (.5 tsp. or to taste)
- Broccoli (1 head)
- Red bell pepper (1)

Prep Technique:
1. Program the cooker using the low heat setting.
2. Slice the steak and into one to two-inch chunks.
3. Pour in the beef broth, aminos, steak, ginger, sweetener, garlic cloves, salt, and red pepper flakes.
4. Cook five to six hours on the low setting.
5. Slice the red pepper into one-inch pieces, and slice the broccoli into florets. After the steak is cooked, stir well.
6. Toss in the peppers and broccoli on top of everything in the slow cooker. Continue cooking for at least one more hour.
7. Add everything together, and sprinkle with sesame seeds for topping.

Cheeseburger Calzone

Servings Provided: 8

Macro Counts Per Serving:
- **Calories**: 580
- **Protein**: 34 g
- **Fat Content**: 47 g
- **Total Net Carbs**: 3 g

Ingredient List:
- Dill pickle spears (4)
- Cream cheese – divided (8 oz.)
- Shredded mozzarella cheese (1 cup)
- Egg (1)
- Yellow diced onion (.5 of 1)
- Ground beef - lean (1.5 lb.)
- Thick-cut bacon strips (4)
- Mayonnaise (.5 cup)
- Shredded cheddar cheese (1 cup)
- Almond flour (1 cup)

Prep Technique:
1. Program the oven temperature setting to 425° Fahrenheit. Prepare a cookie tin with parchment paper.
2. Chop the pickles into spears. Set aside for now.
3. Prepare the crust. Combine about half of the cream cheese and mozzarella cheese. Microwave 35 seconds. When it melts, add the egg and almond flour to make the dough. Set aside.
4. Cook the beef on the stove using the medium heat setting.
5. Prepare the bacon until crunchy (microwave for five minutes or stovetop). When cool, break into bits.
6. Dice the onion and add to the beef. Cook until softened. Toss in the bacon, cheddar cheese, pickle bits, the rest of the cream cheese, and mayonnaise. Stir well.

7. Roll the dough onto the prepared baking tin. Scoop the mixture into the center. Fold the ends and side to make the calzone.
8. Bake until browned or about 15 minutes. Let it rest for 10 minutes before slicing.

Cube Steak- Instant Pot

Servings Provided: 8

Macro Counts Per Serving:
- **Calories**: 154
- **Protein**: 23.5 g
- **Fat Content**: 5.5 g
- **Total Net Carbs**: 3 g

Ingredient List:
- Water (1 cup)
- Cubed steaks(8- 28 oz. pkg.)
- Black pepper (as desired)
- Garlic salt/adobo seasoning (1.75 tsp.)
- Tomato sauce (8 oz. can)
- Green pitted olives (.33 cup) + the brine (2 tbsp.)
- Red pepper (1 small)
- Medium onion (.5 of 1 or 2 small)

Prep Technique:
1. Chop the peppers and onions into ¼-inch strips.
2. Prepare the beef with the salt/adobo and pepper. Toss into the Instant Pot with the remainder of the fixings.
3. Secure the top and prepare for 25 minutes under high pressure. Natural release the pressure and serve.

Oven-Roasted Burgers

Servings Provided: 4

Macro Counts Per Serving:
- **Calories**: 262
- **Protein**: 19 g
- **Fat Content**: 18 g
- **Total Net Carbs**: 4 g

Ingredient List:
- Thinly sliced onion (.5 of 1)
- Ground beef (1 lb.)
- Garlic powder (1 tsp.)
- Black pepper (1 tsp.)
- Onion powder (1 tsp.)
- Salt (1 tsp.)
- American cheese (2 slices)
- *Optional for Serving*: 1 sliced avocado/tomato

Prep Technique:
1. Set the oven to 400° Fahrenheit.
2. Use aluminum foil to cover a baking tin.
3. Combine the beef and seasonings (salt, pepper, onion powder, and garlic powder). Shape into four patties and place them into the pan.
4. Bake one side for ten minutes and flip. Continue cooking until done (ten more minutes) and add the cheese and onions.
5. Cook five more minutes and serve with some tomato or avocado slices. *Note:* The carbs are not calculated into the recipe nutritional information.

Slow-Cooked Steak Tacos

Servings Provided: 4

Macro Counts Per Serving:
- **Calories**: 196
- **Protein**: 25g
- **Fat Content**: 8 g
- **Total Net Carbs**: 4 g

Ingredient List:
- Chopped onion (.5 of 1)
- Bay leaves (1-2)
- Garlic cloves (4)
- Ancho chili powder (1.5 tsp.)
- Smoked paprika (1.5 tsp.)
- Salt and ground black pepper (.5 tsp. each)
- Beef broth (.5 cup)
- Tri-tip roast (1 lb.)

Prep Technique:
1. Remove the fat from the roast.
2. Mince the garlic into a paste using a garlic press or a food processor. You can also use the back of a knife and some coarse sea salt.
3. Combine the salt, pepper, chili powder, and paprika together to form a rub. Coat the meat.
4. Toss in the onions and empty the beef broth into the slow cooker, adding the meat last. Cook eight hours using the low setting.
5. Remove the lid and shred the meat about 30 minutes from the end of the cycle (7.5 hrs.). Leave the cover off to simmer for the last 30 minutes.
6. Serve as a lettuce wrap or other favorite choice.

Stuffed Meatloaf

Servings Provided: 8

Macro Counts Per Serving:
- **Calories**: 248.6
- **Protein**: 15.8 g
- **Fat Content**: 19.56 g
- **Total Net Carbs**: 1.42 g

Ingredient List:
- Cheddar cheese (6 slices)
- Ground beef (1.75 lb.)
- Spinach (.25 cup)
- Mushrooms (.25 cup)
- Green onions (.25 cup)
- Yellow onions (.25 cup)

Ingredient List - As Desired:
- Cumin
- Garlic
- Salt
- Pepper

Prep Technique:
1. Warm the oven to 350° Fahrenheit.
2. Combine the meat with the garlic and spices to your liking.
3. Grease a meatloaf pan. Leave the center open for the stuffing.
4. Chop the onions and combine with the mushrooms and spinach.
5. Mix a portion of the beef over the top with a layer of spinach, and mushrooms (for the top).
6. Bake one hour and enjoy it.

Taco Cabbage Skillet

Servings Provided: 4

Macro Counts Per Serving:
- **Calories**: 325
- **Protein**: 30 g
- **Fat Content**: 21 g
- **Total Net Carbs**: 4 g

Ingredient List:
- Ground beef (1 lb.)
- Salsa - ex. Pace Organic (.5 cup)
- Shredded cabbage (2 cups)
- Chili powder (2 tsp.)
- Shredded cheese (.75 cup)
- Salt and pepper (as desired)
- *Optional Garnishes*: Sour cream and green onions

Prep Technique:
1. Brown the beef and drain the fat. Pour in the salsa, cabbage, and seasoning.
2. Cover and lower the heat. Simmer for 10-12 minutes using the medium heat setting.
3. When the cabbage has softened, extinguish the heat and mix in the cheese.
4. Garnish with your favorite toppings and serve.

Pork and Lamb Options

Grilled Pork Kebabs

Servings Provided: 4
Macro Counts Per Serving:
- **Protein**: 34 g
- **Fat Content**: 9 g
- **Total Net Carbs**: 3.3 g

Ingredient List:
- Hot sauce (2 tsp.)
- Sunflower seed butter (3 tbsp.)
- Minced garlic (1 tbsp.)
- Keto-friendly soy sauce (1 tbsp.)
- Water (1 tbsp.)
- Medium green pepper (1)
- Crushed red pepper (.5 tsp.)
- Squared pork for kebabs (1 lb.)

Prep Technique:
1. Warm up the oven or grill using the broil or the high heat setting.
2. In a processor or blender, combine the water with the red pepper, soy sauce, garlic, butter, and hot sauce.
3. Slice the pork into squares. Cover with the marinade and rest for one hour.
4. Chop the peppers to fit the skewer. Thread the skewers alternating the pork and peppers.
5. Broil using the high heat setting for five minutes per side.

Pork Carnitas - Instant Pot

Servings Provided: 11

Macro Counts Per Serving:
- **Calories**: 160
- **Protein**: 20 g
- **Fat Content**: 7 g
- **Total Net Carbs**: 1 g

Ingredient List:
- Shoulder blade roast (2.5 lb.) trimmed and boneless
- Kosher salt (2 tsp.)
- Black pepper (as desired)
- Cumin (1.5 tsp.)
- Minced garlic (6 cloves)
- Sazon GOYA (.5 tsp.)
- Dried oregano (.25 tsp.)
- Reduced-sodium chicken broth (.75 cup)
- Bay leaves (2)
- Chipotle peppers in adobo sauce (2-3)
- Dry adobo seasoning – ex. Goya (.25 tsp.)
- Garlic powder (.5 tsp.)

Prep Technique:
1. Prepare the roast with pepper and salt. Sear the roast for about five minutes in a skillet. Let it cool and insert the garlic slivers into the roast using a blade (approximately one-inch deep). Season with the garlic powder, sazon, cumin, oregano, and adobo.
2. Arrange the chicken in the Instant Pot, and add the broth, chipotle peppers, and bay leaves. Stir and secure the lid. Prepare using high pressure for 50 minutes (meat button).
3. Natural release the pressure and shred the pork. Combine with the juices, and trash the bay leaves.
4. Add a bit more cumin and adobo if needed. Stir well and serve.

Pork-Chop Fat Bombs

Servings Provided: 3

Macro Counts Per Serving:
- **Calories**: 1076
- **Protein**: 30 g
- **Fat Content**: 103 g
- **Total Net Carbs**: 7 g

Ingredient List:
- Boneless pork chops (3)
- Oil (.5 cup)
- Medium yellow onion (1)
- Brown mushrooms (8 oz.)
- Nutmeg (1 tsp.)
- Garlic powder (1 tsp.)
- Mayonnaise (1 cup)
- Balsamic vinegar (1 tbsp.)

Prep Technique:
1. Rinse, drain, and slice the mushrooms. Peel and slice the onion. Put them in a large skillet with oil and sauté until wilted.
2. Place the chops to the side and sprinkle using the nutmeg and garlic powder. Cook until done.
3. Transfer the prepared chops onto a plate.
4. Whisk the vinegar and mayonnaise in the pan. The thick sauce can be thinned with a bit of chicken broth if needed. (Add 2 tablespoons at a time.)
5. Ladle the sauce over the bomb and serve.

Roasted Leg of Lamb

Servings Provided: 2

Macro Counts Per Serving:
- **Calories**: 223
- **Protein**: 22 g
- **Fat Content**: 14 g
- **Total Net Carbs**: 1 g

Ingredient List:
- Reduced-sodium beef broth (.5 cup)
- Leg of lamb (2 lb.)
- Chopped garlic cloves (6)
- Fresh rosemary leaves (1 tbsp.)
- Black pepper (1 tsp.)
- Salt (2 tsp.)

Prep Technique:
1. Grease a baking pan and set the oven temperature to 400° Fahrenheit.
2. Arrange the lamb in the pan and add the broth and seasonings.
3. Roast 30 minutes and lower the heat to 350° Fahrenheit.
4. Continue cooking for about one hour or until done.
5. Let the lamb stand about 20 minutes before slicing to serve.
6. Enjoy with some roasted brussels sprouts and extra rosemary for a tasty change of pace.

Seafood

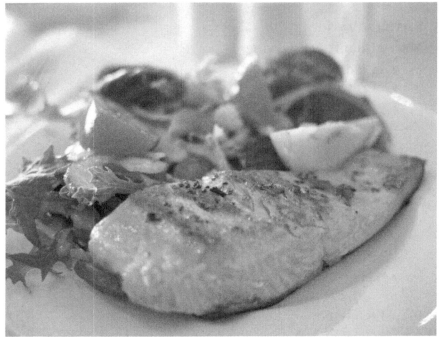

Asian Style Tuna Patties

Servings Provided: 6

Macro Counts Per Serving:
- **Calories**: 145
- **Protein**: 17.7 g
- **Fat Content**: 4.2 g
- **Total Net Carbs**: 3.8 g

Ingredient List:
- Light tuna (2 cans)
- Sesame oil (1 tsp.)
- Keto-friendly bread - reduced-calorie (2 slices) or dried breadcrumbs (.75 cup)
- Egg substitute - ex. Eggbeaters (.25 cup)
- Garlic (1 clove)
- Green onions (3)

- Black pepper (1 tsp.)
- Teriyaki sauce (1 tbsp.)
- Ketchup (1 tbsp.)
- Soy sauce (1 tbsp.)
- Cooking oil spray (as needed)

Prep Technique:

1. Prepare the breadcrumbs. Bake the slices of bread at 200° Fahrenheit until dried out. Put in a blender or food processor to equal ¾ cup.
2. Drain the tuna. Peel and mince the garlic and onions. Mix the egg, tuna, breadcrumbs, garlic, and green onions in a large bowl.
3. Blend the teriyaki sauce, soy sauce, ketchup, pepper, and sesame oil into the mixture.
4. Shape the tuna patties into a one-inch thickness.
5. Over medium heat in a greased pan with a bit of nonstick cooking spray, fry each side for approximately 5 minutes.
6. Serve with your favorite side dish.

Baked Tilapia and Cherry Tomatoes

Servings Provided: 2

Macro Counts Per Serving:

- **Calories**: 180
- **Protein**: 23 g
- **Fat Content**: 8 g
- **Total Net Carbs**: 4 g

Ingredient List:

- Butter (2 tsp.)
- Tilapia fillets (2 - 4 oz.)
- Cherry tomatoes (8)
- Pitted black olives (.25 cup)
- Garlic powder (1 tsp.)
- Black pepper (.25 tsp.)
- Paprika (.25 tsp.)
- Salt (.5 tsp.)
- Freshly squeezed lemon juice (1 tbsp.)
- *Optional:* Balsamic vinegar (1 tbsp.)

Prep Technique:

1. Set the oven to reach 375 ° Fahrenheit.
2. Grease a roasting pan and add the butter along with the olives and tomatoes at the bottom.
3. Season the tilapia with the spices (paprika, salt, pepper, and garlic powder). Lastly, add the fish fillets lemon juice.
4. Cover the pan with foil and bake until

Ginger and Sesame Salmon

Servings Provided: 2

Macro Counts Per Serving:

- **Calories**: 370
- **Protein**: 33 g
- **Fat Content**: 23.5 g
- **Total Net Carbs**: 2.5 g

Ingredient List:

- Salmon fillet (1 - 10 oz.)
- Sesame oil (2 tsp.)
- White wine 2 tbsp.)
- Soy sauce (2 tbsp.)
- Minced ginger (1-2 tsp.)
- Rice vinegar (1 tbsp.)
- Sugar-free ketchup (1 tbsp.)
- Fish sauce – ex. Red Boat (1 tbsp.)

Prep Technique:

1. Combine all of the fixings in a plastic container with a tight-fitting lid (omit the ketchup, oil, and wine for now). Marinade them for about 1o to 15 minutes.
2. On the stovetop, prepare a skillet over high heat and pour in the oil. Add the fish when it's hot, skin side down.
3. Brown both sides for three to four minutes.
4. Add the marinated juices to the pan and let it simmer when the fish is flipped. Arrange the fish on two dinner plates.
5. Pour in the wine and ketchup to the pan and simmer five minutes until it's reduced. Serve with your favorite vegetable.

Lemon and Dill Wild-Caught Salmon - Slow-Cooked

Servings Provided: 4

Macro Counts Per Serving:

- **Calories**: 341
- **Protein**: 50 g
- **Fat Content**: 13 g
- **Total Net Carbs**: 2 g

Ingredient List:

- Water (2 cups)
- Wild-caught skin-on salmon (2 lb.)
- Reduced-sodium vegetable broth (1 cup)
- Finely chopped onion (1)
- Thinly sliced lemon (1)
- Pepper and salt (as desired)
- Dill sprigs (3)

Prep Technique:

1. Combine all of the fixings in a slow cooker, with the salmon on the bottom.
2. Prepare using the high setting for two hours. It's done once it flakes easily.

Miso Salmon

Servings Provided: 4

Macro Counts Per Serving:
- **Calories**: 215
- **Protein**: 28.38 g
- **Fat Content**: 9.23 g
- **Total Net Carbs**: 0.78 g

Ingredient List:
- Salmon fillets – skin-on (1.25 lb.)
- White wine (2 tbsp.)
- Sake (3 tbsp.)
- Miso – White suggested (3 tbsp.)
- Kosher salt (as desired)

Prep Technique:
1. Slice the salmon into fillets and sprinkle with the salt. Rest for 30 minutes to help remove some of the moisture. Gently wipe off the salt with a towel with 1 tbsp. of the sake.
2. Mix the white wine, miso, and the rest of the sake in a dish.
3. Pour approximately 1/3 of the marinade in an airtight bowl. Add the fillets and add the rest of the marinade. Refrigerate for 1 to 2 days.
4. When ready to eat, warm up the oven to 400° Fahrenheit. Cover a baking tin with parchment paper.
5. Scrape away the marinade with your fingers to help prevent burning.
6. Bake 25 minutes and serve.

Zucchini Lasagna With Tofu Ricotta and Walnut Sauce

Servings Provided: 4
Macro Counts Per Serving:
- **Calories**: 356
- **Protein**: 17 g
- **Fat Content**: 25 g
- **Total Net Carbs**: 10 g

Ingredient List - The Sauce:
- Walnuts - finely ground (1 cup)
- Marinara sauce (divided - 1 jar or 25 oz.)
- Chopped sun-dried tomatoes (.25 cup)

Ingredient List - The Lasagna:
- Zucchini (2)
- Tofu Ricotta (1 batch)
- Nutritional Yeast - optional (2 tbsp.)

Ingredient List - The Ricotta:
- Minced garlic (1 clove)
- Firm tofu (14 oz. firm drained and pressed)
- Olive oil (1 tbsp.)
- Dried basil (1 tbsp.)
- Nutritional yeast (3 tbsp.)
- Lemon juice (1 tbsp.)
- Pepper and salt (as desired)

Prep Technique:
1. Warm up the oven to 375° Fahrenheit.
2. Slice the zucchini with a mandolin (11-inches lengthwise).
3. Prepare the ricotta by pulsing all of the fixings in a food processor until creamy smooth.
4. Combine the marinara and walnuts with the sun-dried tomatoes - reserving ¾ cup for the pan.

5. Prepare a baking pan 7.5x9.5 and add the reserved sauce with a layer of zucchini. Spread the tofu ricotta over the noodles followed by a sprinkle of the yeast. Pour about half the walnut sauce on the top
6. Layer until finished and bake for 35 minutes until done.

Bread Option

Dinner Rolls

Servings Provided: 6 rolls
Macro Counts Per Serving:
- **Calories**: 219
- **Protein**: 10.7 g
- **Fat Content**: 18 g
- **Total Net Carbs**: 2.3 g

Ingredient List:
- Mozzarella (1 cup - shredded)
- Cream cheese (1 oz.)
- Almond flour (1 cup)
- Ground flaxseed (.25 cup)
- Egg (1)
- Baking soda (.5 tsp.)

Prep Technique:
1. Warm the oven to reach 400° Fahrenheit.
2. Line a baking tin with a sheet of parchment baking paper.
3. Melt the mozzarella and cream cheese together (microwave for 1 min.).
4. Stir well and add a whisked egg. Combine well.
5. In another container, whisk the baking soda, almond flour, and flaxseed. Mix in the cheese mixture to form a sticky soft-ball.
6. Wet your hands slightly and roll the dough into six balls.
7. Roll the tops of the rolls in sesame seeds and place them on the baking sheet.
8. Bake until nicely browned (10-12 min.).
9. Cool 15 minutes and serve.

Chapter 6: Scrumptious Desserts

Apple Crisp With Blackberries

Servings Provided: 8

Macro Counts Per Serving:
- **Calories**: 200
- **Protein**: 3 g
- **Fat Content**: 16 g
- **Total Net Carbs**: 13 g

Ingredient List - The Topping:
- Chopped pecans (.5 cup)
- Blanched almond flour (.5 cup)
- Confectioners swerve sweetener (.25 cup)
- Salted butter (3 tbsp. melted)
- Ground cinnamon (.5 tsp.)

Ingredient List - The Filling:
- Golden delicious apples (3 small)
- Fresh blackberries (1.25 cups)
- Confectioners swerve sweetener (.25 cup)
- Water (.25 cup)
- Salted butter (2 tbsp.)
- Ground cinnamon (1 tbsp.)
- Vanilla extract (1 tsp.)
- *Also Needed:* Glass 1.5-quart - 9×5-inch loaf pan and a 10-inch nonstick skillet

Prep Technique:
1. Peel and core the apples into eight wedges. Position an oven rack in the center of the oven. Preheat to 350° Fahrenheit.
2. Make the Topping: In a large mixing bowl, add all topping ingredients except the melted butter, stirring until well-

mixed. Add butter and continue stirring until its appearance is that of moistened crumbles. Set aside.

3. Prepare the Filling: In a skillet, melt butter using medium heat. As it starts to bubble, stir occasionally to avoid burning. Carefully stir in water to cool the butter, adding in the sweetener, cinnamon, and vanilla until dissolved.

4. Bring to a simmer, and add the apple wedges and blackberries. Cook until most of the released liquid is evaporated, and the softened apples are easily punctured (10 to 15 min.), stirring frequently for even cooking. Turn off the heat.

5. Transfer the filling to a loaf baking dish, spreading out the filling to cover the bottom of the dish. Spread the topping over the filling, breaking up large chunks and making sure the filling is covered by the topping.

6. Transfer the dish to the oven, baking until the topping looks crisp (15 to 20 min.). Let it cool for about 10 minutes before serving.

7. *Note:* Use sweet and crisp varieties such as golden delicious, Honeycrisp, or Braeburn, which better maintain their texture and shape during cooking.

Blueberry Cupcakes

Servings Provided: 12

Macro Counts Per Serving:
- **Calories**: 138
- **Protein**: 4.4 g
- **Fat Content**: 11.4 g
- **Total Net Carbs**: 2.8 g

Ingredient List:
- Melted butter (1 stick)
- Coconut flour (.5 cup)
- Granulated sweetener of choice (4 tbsp.)
- Baking powder (1 tsp.)
- Lemon juice (2 tbsp.)
- Vanilla (1 tsp.)
- Zest of a lemon (2 tbsp.)
- Eggs (8 medium)
- Fresh blueberries (1 cup)
- *Also Needed:* 12-cupcake holder and liners

Prep Technique:
1. Set the oven temperature to 350° Fahrenheit.
2. Combine the melted butter, sweetener, coconut flour, baking powder, vanilla, lemon juice, and zest together.
3. Whisk the eggs, adding them in one at a time. Mix well.
4. Taste the cupcake batter to ensure you have used enough sweetener and flavors to mask the subtle taste of coconut from the coconut flour.
5. Dump the batter into the tins.
6. Press in a few fresh blueberries in the batter of each cupcake.
7. Pop into the oven to bake until golden brown or about 15 minutes.
8. Cover with sugar-free cream cheese frosting. Vanilla or lemon flavor is perfect. Garnish with fresh blueberries and lemon zest.
9. *Note*: Icing/frosting is additional and optional.

Chocolate-Filled Peanut Butter Cookies

Servings Provided: 20

Macro Counts Per Serving:
- **Calories**: 150
- **Protein**: 4.5 g
- **Fat Content**: 14 g
- **Total Net Carbs**: 2.7 g

Ingredient List:
- Almond flour (2.5 cups)
- Peanut butter (.5 cup)
- Coconut oil (.25 cup)
- Erythritol (.25 cup)
- Maple syrup (3 tbsp.)
- Vanilla extract (1 tbsp.)
- Baking powder (1.5 tsp.)
- Salt (.5 tsp.)
- Dark chocolate bars (2-3)

Prep Technique:
1. Prepare the cookie pan with the paper.
2. Warm up the oven to reach 350° Fahrenheit.
3. Whisk each of the wet fixings together and mix in with the dry ingredients.
4. Mix well and place in the fridge for 20 to 30 minutes.
5. Break the bars into small squares. Shape the dough into little balls until they are flat.
6. Add one to two pieces of chocolate and seal it into the ball.
7. Arrange on the cookie sheet.
8. Bake for about 15 minutes. Remove and serve.

Creamy Lime Pie

Servings Provided: 8

Macro Counts Per Serving:
- **Calories**: 386
- **Protein**: 7 g
- **Fat Content**: 38.6 g
- **Total Net Carbs**: 4.2 g

Ingredient List:
- Melted butter (.25 cup)
- Almond flour (1.5 cups)
- Erythritol (divided - .5 cup)
- Salt (.5 tsp.)
- Heavy cream (1 cup)
- Egg yolks (4)
- Freshly squeezed key lime juice (.33 cup)
- Lime zest (1 tbsp.)
- Cubed cold butter (.25 cup)
- Vanilla extract (1 tsp.)
- Xanthan gum (.25 tsp.)
- Sour cream (1 cup)
- Cream cheese (.5 cup)

Prep Technique:
1. Warm the oven to reach350° Fahrenheit.
2. Melt the butter in a pan.
3. Mix the salt, half or .25 cup of erythritol, and almond flour.
4. Slowly add the butter. Blend and press into a pie platter.
5. Bake for 15 minutes. Remove when it's lightly browned. Let it cool.
6. In another saucepan, combine the egg yolks, heavy cream, lime zest, juice, and the remainder of the erythritol.
7. Simmer using the medium heat temperature setting until it starts to thicken (7-10 min.).

8. Take the pan from the heat and add the xanthan gum, vanilla extract, cold butter, cream cheese, and sour cream. Whisk until smooth.
9. Scoop into the cooled pie shell. Cover and place in the fridge.
10. *Note:* You can serve after four hours, but it is better if you wait overnight to enjoy it.

Dark Chocolate Milkshake

Servings Provided: 2

Macro Counts Per Serving:
- **Calories**: 302
- **Protein**: 4.8 g
- **Fat Content**: 27.1 g
- **Total Net Carbs**: 2.5 g

Ingredient List:
- Heavy whipping cream (6 tbsp.)
- Canned coconut milk (5 tbsp.)
- Vanilla extract (.125 tsp.)
- Unsweetened dark cocoa powder (2 tbsp.)
- Stevia sugar substitute or other sugar substitutes (2 tbsp.)

Prep Technique:
1. Use an electric mixer to prepare the cream. Once stiff peaks have formed, add in the rest of the fixings and continue mixing until stiff peaks form again.
2. Put the mixture into the freezer for about 20 minutes.
3. Take the container out of the freezer and stir. Continue the process until you have reached the desired consistency.

Peanut Butter Cups

Servings Provided: 12

Macro Counts Per Serving:
- **Calories**: 220
- **Protein**: 6 g
- **Fat Content**: 20 g
- **Total Net Carbs**: 2 g

Ingredient List:
- Low-carb milk chocolate (12 oz.)

Ingredient List - Peanut butter mixture:

- Keto-friendly organic peanut butter (3.5 oz.)
- Powdered erythritol (2 tbsp.)
- Whey protein powder (1 oz.)

Prep Technique:
1. Prepare a 12-count muffin tin with paper wrappers.
2. Mix the peanut butter fixings thoroughly, until it becomes a dough that doesn't stick to the sides of the bowl. For easier handling, refrigerate to use later.
3. Melt the chocolate in a double boiler using low heat. Remove from heat once liquid. Pour about 1 tablespoonful into each of the holders.
4. Chill in the refrigerator until firm (15 min.).
5. Take the wrappers and peanut butter out of the refrigerator.
6. Place a .5 tablespoon ball of peanut butter in each wrapper and flatten until it nearly touches the edge of the wrapper.
7. Stir the remaining liquid chocolate and then pour 4 teaspoonsful of chocolate over each filled wrapper.
8. Chill in the fridge until hardened or for about 30 minutes.
9. Store at room temperature.

Peanut Butter Pie

Servings Provided:

Macro Counts Per Serving:
- **Calories**: 430
- **Protein**: 8.1 g
- **Fat Content**: 37.4 g
- **Total Net Carbs**: 7.5 g

Ingredient List - The Chocolate Almond Crust:
- Almond flour (1.5 cups)
- Cocoa (.33 cup)
- Sweetener - swerve (.25 cup)
- Melted butter (5 tbsp.)

Ingredient List - The Filling:
- Unchilled cream cheese (24 oz.)
- Smooth, natural peanut butter (.75 cup)
- Pyure Organic Stevia Blend sweetener (.75 cup)
- Whipping cream (1.5 cups)
- Cream of tartar (.5 tsp.)

Prep Technique:
1. Unchill the cream cheese on the countertop for about two hours before you begin.
2. Prepare the crust. Mix and press into a springform 9-inch pan and bake at 400° Fahrenheit for 8-10 minutes.
3. In another container, whisk the sweetener and whipping cream. Mix in the cream of tartar.
4. In another mixing container, combine the cream cheese and nut butter.
5. Combine the mixtures and fill the pan into the crust.
6. Chill for 30-45 minutes in the freezer or for 3 to 4 hours in the fridge
7. Dust with crushed peanuts and cocoa before serving.

Pecan Pie Clusters

Servings Provided: 10 clusters
Macro Counts Per Serving:
- **Calories**: 140
- **Protein**: 1 g
- **Fat Content**: 14 g
- **Total Net Carbs**: 1 g

Ingredient List:
- Chopped pecans (1 cup)
- Dark or sugar-free chocolate (2 oz. - chopped)
- Butter (3 tbsp.)
- Heavy cream (.25 cup)
- Zen Sweet or sweetener of choice (2 tbsp.)
- Vanilla (1 tsp.)

Prep Technique:
1. Using the medium temperature setting, brown the butter until golden. Stir frequently.
2. Once golden, add heavy cream and whisk together. Turn down heat to a simmer. Whisk in the sweetener and vanilla, working until it's lump-free.
3. Whisk occasionally for the next five minutes. (The mixture will have a consistency similar to caramel and slightly darken.) Remove from the heat.
4. Mix in the chopped pecans and spoon the clusters onto a parchment-lined tray. Place in the freezer for five minutes.
5. Microwave dark chocolate for 20-40 seconds until melted and smooth. Drizzle over the clusters and enjoy.

Pumpkin Cheesecake

Servings Provided: 12

Macro Counts Per Serving:
- **Calories**: 346
- **Protein**: 6 g
- **Fat Content**: 33 g
- **Total Net Carbs**: 4 g

Ingredient List - Walnut Crust:
- Walnuts (2 cups)
- Butter, melted (3 tbsp.)
- Cinnamon (1 tsp.)
- Vanilla (.5 tsp.)
- *Optional:* Sweetener (2 tsp.)

Ingredient List - Cheesecake Fluff:
- Cream cheese (16 oz. - softened)
- Powdered swerve (1 cup)
- Heavy whipping cream (.66 cup)
- Pumpkin puree (.66 cup)
- Pumpkin spice (2 tsp.)
- Vanilla (1 tsp.)

Prep Technique:
1. Warm the oven to 350° Fahrenheit.
2. Combine all of the crust fixings in a food processor until it has a dough-like consistency, scraping down the sides as needed.
3. Press the dough into a 9-inch round baking dish. Bake for 12-15 minutes until lightly brown.
4. Remove and let cool for 20 minutes.
5. Prepare the pumpkin fluff. In a large bowl, whip softened cream cheese, heavy whipping cream and swerve together until fluffy (hand mixer or stand mixers works best)
6. Add the pumpkin puree, pumpkin spice, and vanilla. Beat until combined.

7. Spread cheesecake fluff on the cooled walnut crust and refrigerate until set or for at least two hours.

Walnut Cookies

Servings Provided: 16

Macro Counts Per Serving:
- **Calories**: 72
- **Protein**: 3 g
- **Fat Content**: 6.7 g
- **Total Net Carbs**: 1.1 g

Ingredient List:
- Egg (1)
- Ground cinnamon (1 tsp.)
- Erythritol (2 tbsp.)
- Ground walnuts (1.5cups)

Prep Technique:
1. Warm the oven to reach 350° Fahrenheit. Prepare a baking tin with a sheet of parchment baking paper.
2. Combine the cinnamon and erythritol with the egg. Fold in the walnuts.
3. Shape into balls and bake for 10 to 13 minutes. Cool slightly and serve.

Zucchini Spiced Cupcakes

Servings Provided: 12

Macro Counts Per Serving:
- **Calories**: 68
- **Protein**: 4.9 g
- **Fat Content**: 23.1 g
- **Total Net Carbs**: 3.5 g

Ingredient List- The Cakes:
- Almond flour (1 cup)
- Coconut flour (.33 - .5 cup)
- Xanthan gum (.5 tsp.)
- Bak. soda (1 tsp.)
- Bak. powder (.5 tsp.)
- Salt (.5 tsp.)
- Cinnamon (1 tsp.)
- Ground cloves (.125 tsp.)
- Nutmeg (.25 tsp.)
- Coconut oil liquefied (.5 cup)
- Large eggs (2 unchilled)
- Sugar-free vanilla extract (1.5 tsp.)
- Monk fruit sweetener (1 cup)
- Packed grated zucchini (1.5 cups)
- *Optional:* Walnuts coarsely chopped

Ingredient List - The Frosting:
- Softened cream cheese (4 oz.)
- Butter (2 tbsp. softened)
- Monk fruit sweetener - powdered (.5 cup)
- Vanilla extract (.5 tsp.)
- *Also Needed*: Electric mixer or food processor

Prep Technique:
1. Warm the oven in advance to reach 350° Fahrenheit.
2. Sift both flours together. Prepare the muffin tins with paper or foil baking liners.

3. Stir in both types of flour with the baking soda, xanthan gum, baking powder, nutmeg, cinnamon, salt, and cloves. Set aside for now.
4. Whisk the coconut oil, eggs, and vanilla extract. Stir in zucchini and sweetener, and the flour mixture. Fold in the walnuts. Add the batter to the liners.
5. Bake until the cake is firm to touch (25-30 min.).
6. Remove cool on a rack. Frost with cream cheese frosting if desired.
7. Store cupcakes in the refrigerator or freezer.
8. Cool to reach room temperature before serving.

Preparation Steps - The Frosting:
1. Pour the sweetener in a blender.
2. Mix the butter and cream cheese until fully incorporated.
3. Add the vanilla and frost the cake.

Fat Bombs

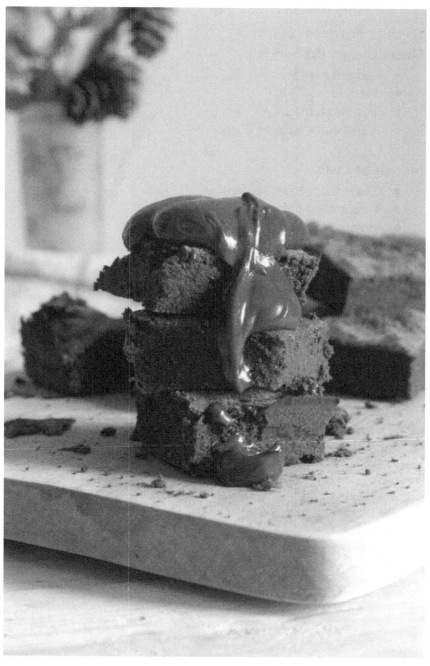

Blueberry Cream Cheese Bombs

Servings Provided: 24

Macro Counts Per Serving:

- **Calories**: 116
- **Protein**: .44 g
- **Fat Content**: 13 g
- **Total Net Carbs**: 1.02 g

Ingredient List:

- Scant blueberries (1 cup)
- Coconut oil (.75 cup)
- Butter (1 stick)
- Coconut cream (.25 cup)
- Softened cream cheese (4 oz.)
- Sweetener of choice

Prep Technique:

1. Arrange three or four berries in each mold cup.
2. Melt the coconut oil and butter over the lowest stovetop heat setting. Cool slightly for approximately five minutes.
3. Combine all of the ingredients and whisk well. Slowly, add the sweetener.
4. Using a spouted pitcher, fill an ice tray with 24 bombs.
5. Pop them out and eat when hunger strikes.

Chocolate Chip Cheesecake Fat Bombs

Servings Provided: 12

Macro Counts Per Serving:

- **Calories**: 112
- **Protein**: 1 g
- **Fat Content**: 12 g
- **Total Net Carbs**: 1 g

Ingredient List:

- Unchilled cream cheese - softened (4 oz.)
- Melted butter (4 tbsp.)
- Coconut oil (.25 cup)
- Sweetener ex. LakantoMonkfruit (2 tbsp.)
- Chocolate chips- ex. Lily's sweetened with stevia (.25 cup)
- Vanilla extract (1 tsp.)

Prep Technique:

1. Prepare a mini cupcake pan with or without liners
2. Combine the melted butter, cream cheese, coconut oil, sweetener, and vanilla extract in a mixing container.
3. Using a hand mixer, blend for two to three minutes until smooth.
4. Fold in the chocolate chips, holding a few to add as a garnish to each bomb as desired.
5. Scoop the mixture into the muffin tin.
6. Freeze for 30 minutes. Remove from the tray and serve.

Cocoa Butter Walnut Fat Bombs

Servings Provided: 8
Macro Counts Per Serving:
- **Calories**: 265
- **Protein**: 0.9 g
- **Fat Content**: 20 g
- **Total Net Carbs**: 0.3 g

Ingredient List:
- Coconut oil (4 tbsp.)
- Erythritol (4 tbsp. powdered)
- Butter (4 tbsp.)
- Cocoa butter (4 oz.)
- Chopped walnuts (.5 cup)
- Vanilla extract (.5 tsp.)
- Salt (.25 tsp)

Prep Technique:
1. Prepare a pan using the medium-high temperature setting on the stovetop. Add the butter, coconut oil, and cocoa butter.
2. Once it's melted, add the walnuts, salt, stevia, vanilla extract, and erythritol. Mix well.
3. Pour into the silicone mold. Store the treats in the refrigerator for one hour before serving.

Lemon Cheesecake Fat Bombs

Servings Provided: 16

Macro Counts Per Serving:
- **Calories**: 60
- **Protein**: 1 g
- **Fat Content**: 7 g
- **Total Net Carbs**: 0.5 g

Ingredient List:
- Cream cheese (6 oz. - note that each brick is 8 oz.)
- Salted butter (4 tbsp.)
- Granular swerve sweetener (1.5 oz. /3 tbsp.)
- Fresh lemon juice (2 tbsp.)
- *Optional*: Finely grated lemon zest (1 tbsp.)
- *Also Needed*: Silicone molds

Prep Technique:
1. Let the cream cheese and butter sit at room temperature until softened before continuing with the recipe.
2. Whisk the sweetener, lemon juice, and lemon zest. Whisk until well-mixed.
3. In another bowl, microwave the cream cheese until very soft (10 sec.).
4. Add the cream cheese and butter to the bowl with the lemon juice mixture. Use an electric hand mixer (low speed) to beat until well-mixed.
5. Divide the batter into the molds. Freeze for several hours until solid before serving.
6. Store the leftovers in the freezer.

Orange and Walnut Chocolate Fat Bombs

Servings Provided: 8
Macro Counts Per Serving:
- **Calories**: 87
- **Protein**: 1 g
- **Fat Content**: 9 g
- **Total Net Carbs**: 2 g

Ingredient List:
- 85% Cocoa dark chocolate (12.5 grams)
- Extra-Virgin coconut oil (.25 cup)
- Orange peel or orange extract (.5 tbsp.)
- Walnuts (1.75 cups)
- Cinnamon (1 tsp.)
- Stevia (10-15 drops)

Prep Technique:
1. Use the microwave, or a saucepan to melt the chocolate. Add cinnamon and coconut oil. Sweeten mixture with stevia.
2. Pour in the fresh orange peel and chopped walnuts.
3. In a muffin tin or in candy mold, spoon in the mixture.
4. Place in the refrigerator for one to three hours until the mixture is solid.

Chapter 7: Healthy Snack Options

Almond Coconut Bars

Servings Provided: 6
Macro Counts Per Serving:
- **Calories**: 253
- **Protein**: 5 g
- **Fat Content**: 25 g
- **Total Net Carbs**: 2 g

Ingredient List:
- Coconut oil (.5 cup)
- Almond flour (1.25 cups)
- Coconut flour (.25 cup
- Eggs (2)
- Sugar substitute (3 tbsp.)
- Almond butter (2 tbsp.)
- Salt (.25 tsp.)
- Water (1 cup)
- Vanilla extract (1 tsp.)
- *Also Needed:* Baking pan and Trivet for the Instant Pot

Prep Technique:
1. Line the pan that fits in the cooker with the baking paper.
2. Combine all of the fixings in the food processor. Empty into the pan.
3. Empty the water into the Instant Pot with the steamer rack. Arrange the pan in the cooker and secure the lid.
4. Set the timer for 15 minutes.
5. Natural-release the pressure and chill the pan until its room temperature.
6. Slice into six bars.

Bacon Guacamole Fat Bombs

Servings Provided: 6

Macro Counts Per Serving:

- **Calories**: 156
- **Protein**: 3.4 g
- **Fat Content**: 15.2 g
- **Total Net Carbs**: 1.4 g

Ingredient List:

- Avocado (.5 of large or 3.5 oz.)
- Bacon (4 strips)
- Butter or ghee (.25 cup)
- Garlic cloves (2 crushed)
- Diced onion (.5 of 1 small)
- Finely chopped chili pepper (1 small)
- Fresh lime juice (1 tbsp.)
- Salt (to your liking)
- Ground black pepper or cayenne (1 pinch)
- Freshly chopped cilantro (1-2 tbsp.)

Prep Technique:

1. Program the oven setting to 375° Fahrenheit.
2. Line the tray with parchment paper and cook the bacon for ten to fifteen minutes. Save the grease for step four.
3. Peel, deseed, and chop the avocado into a dish along with the garlic, chili pepper, lime juice, cilantro, black pepper, salt, and butter.
4. Use a fork or potato masher to combine the mixture and blend in the onion.
5. Empty the grease into the bomb, blend well, and cover for 20 to 30 minutes in the refrigerator. Make six balls.
6. Break up the bacon into a bowl and roll the balls in it until coated evenly and serve for breakfast or a snack.

Baked Apples

Servings Provided: 4

Macro Counts Per Serving:
- **Calories**: 175
- **Protein**: 7 g
- **Fat Content**: 20 g
- **Total Net Carbs**: 16g

Ingredient List:
- Keto-friendly sweetener (4 tsp. or to taste)
- Cinnamon (.75 tsp.)
- Chopped pecans (.25 cup)
- Granny Smith apples (4 large)

Prep Technique:
1. Set the oven temperature at 375° Fahrenheit.
2. Mix the sweetener with the cinnamon and pecans.
3. Core the apple and add the prepared stuffing.
4. Add enough water into the baking dish to cover the bottom of the apple.
5. Bake for about 45 minutes to 1 hour.

Chocolate Dipped Candied Bacon

Servings Provided: 16

Macro Counts Per Serving:
- **Calories**: 54
- **Protein**: 3 g
- **Fat Content**: 4.1 g
- **Total Net Carbs**: 1.1 g

Ingredient List:
- Thin-cut slices of bacon (16)
- Brown sugar alternative – ex. Sukrin Gold or erythritol (2 tbsp.)
- Cinnamon (.5 tsp.)
- Cacao butter (.5 oz.) or coconut oil (1 tbsp.)
- 85% dark chocolate (3 oz.)
- Sugar-free maple extract (1 tsp.)

Prep Technique:
1. Mix the *Sukrin Gold* sweetener with the cinnamon.
2. Lay the strips of bacon onto a parchment paper-lined tray. Sprinkle with half of the mixture.
3. Turn them over and do the other side with the rest of the mix.
4. Heat up the oven to reach 275° Fahrenheit. Bake until caramelized and crispy (60 to 75 min.).
5. Warm a pan to melt the cocoa butter and chocolate. Pour the maple syrup into the mixture and stir well. Set to the side until it's room temperature.
6. Arrange the bacon on a platter to cool thoroughly before dipping into the chocolate.
7. Dip half of each strip of bacon in the chocolate. Place on a tray for the chocolate to solidify. You can place it in the fridge or just on the countertop.

Cinnamon Vanilla Protein Bites

Servings Provided: 18-20 bites

Macro Counts Per Serving:

- **Calories**: 112
- **Protein**: 2 g
- **Fat Content**: 9 g
- **Total Net Carbs**: 4 g

Ingredient List:

- Quick oats (.75 cup)
- Nut butter of choice (.25 - .33 cup)
- Cinnamon (1 tbsp.)
- Pure maple syrup (.25 - .33 cup)
- Vanilla protein powder (.25 cup)
- Almond meal (.5 cup)
- Vanilla extract (.5 - 1 tsp.)
- *Also Needed:* Food processor

Prep Technique:

1. Line a cookie tin with a layer of parchment paper.
2. Grind the oats with the processor and add to a mixing container. Combine the cinnamon, protein powder, almond meal, and nut butter.
3. Mix in the syrup and vanilla. Using your hands, mix well, and roll into small balls.
4. Freeze for 20 to 30 minutes.
5. Store in a Ziploc-type baggie with the cinnamon and vanilla protein mixture.

Guacamole Deviled Eggs

Servings Provided: 8

Macro Counts Per Serving:
- **Calories**: 119
- **Protein**: 4.2g
- **Fat Content**: 9.9 g
- **Total Net Carbs**: 5g

Ingredient List:
- Eggs (4 in the shell)
- Minced green onion (1 tbsp.)
- Chopped cilantro (1 tbsp.)
- Avocados (2 peeled, pitted, and mashed)
- Fresh lime juice (2 tsp.)
- Seeded jalapeno pepper (2 tsp.)
- Hot pepper sauce (dash Tabasco)
- Salt (.5 tsp.)
- Dijon-style mustard (1 tsp.)
- Worcestershire sauce (1 tsp.)
- Paprika (1 pinch)

Prep Technique:
1. Gently arrange the eggs in a saucepan – covered with clean water. Place a lid on the pot, and let it simmer for 10-12 minutes.
2. Transfer the eggs from the pot and let them cool in a container of cold water. When chilled, slice into halves and add the yolks to a mixing container. Toss in the cilantro, avocado, jalapeno, and onion.
3. Stir in the juice along with the mustard, Worcestershire sauce, salt, and hot sauce. Blend well.
4. Fill the egg white halves and stick in the fridge until ready to eat.
5. Sprinkle using the paprika.

Spicy Deviled Eggs

Servings Provided: 6

Macro Counts Per Serving:

- **Calories**: 200
- **Protein**: 6 g
- **Fat Content**: 19 g
- **Total Net Carbs**: 1 g

Ingredient List:

- Eggs (6)
- Mayonnaise (.5 cup)
- Red curry paste (1 tbsp.)
- Poppy seeds (.5 tbsp.)
- Salt (.25 tsp.)

Prep Technique:

1. Prepare a pan with just enough water to cover the eggs. Do *not* put a lid on the pot but bring it to a boil.
2. Cook the eggs for about 8 minutes. Place into an ice water bath at that time.
3. Discard the eggshells and cut the eggs in half. Scoop out the egg yolk.
4. Place the whites on a platter and place it in the fridge.
5. Combine the mayonnaise, curry paste, and egg yolks until smooth.
6. Take the egg whites from the fridge and apply the prepared yolks. Sprinkle with the seeds on top to serve.

Chapter 8: 28-Day Meal Plan

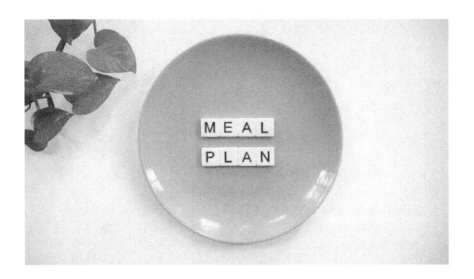

This is your special meal plan to get you started on the ketogenic journey. Each one has been calculated with minimal carbs, so you still have some flexibility for other special options on the keto plan for each day no matter which intermittent fasting plan you choose.

Day 1:
Breakfast: Chocolate Pecan Pie and Muffins (3.4 g)
Lunch: Swedish Dill Shrimp Salad (2 g)
Dinner: Pork-Chop Fat Bombs (7 g)
Snack or Dessert: Cinnamon Vanilla Protein Bites (4 g)

Day 2:
Breakfast: Single-Serve Baked Eggs (0.6 g)
Lunch: Asiago Tomato Soup (8.75 g)
Dinner: Oven-Roasted Burgers (4 g)
Snack or Dessert: Dark Chocolate Milkshake (2.5 g)

Day 3:

Breakfast: Blueberry Kefir Smoothie (6.6 g)
Lunch: Slow-Cooked Teriyaki (4 g)
Dinner: Lemon and Dill Wild-Caught Salmon - Slow-Cooked (2 g) and
>   Dinner Rolls (2.3 g)
Snack or Dessert: Peanut Butter Pie (7.5 g)

Day 4:
Breakfast: Brunch Ham Rolls (7.2 g)
Lunch: Loaded Cauliflower Bowl (3 g)
Dinner: Balsamic Chicken Thighs (3.6 g)
Snack or Dessert: Pumpkin Cheesecake (4 g)

Day 5:
Breakfast: Banana Avocado Muffins (4 g)
Lunch: No Beans Beef Chili (5 g)
Dinner: Zucchini Lasagna With Tofu Ricotta and Walnut Sauce (10 g)
Snack or Dessert: Almond Coconut Bars (2 g)

Day 6:
Breakfast: Carrot Cake Pancakes (5 g)
Lunch: Bacon and Shrimp Risotto (5.3 g)
Dinner: Taco Cabbage Skillet (4 g)
Snack or Dessert: Blueberry Cupcakes (2.8 g)

Day 7:
Breakfast: Bacon Baked Denver Omelet (3.6 g)
Lunch: Shrimp Avocado Salad With Tomatoes and Feta (6.5 g)
Dinner: Cube Steak- Instant Pot (3 g)
Snack or Dessert: Pecan Pie Clusters (1 g)

Day 8:
Breakfast: Cinnamon Raisin Bagels (6 g)
Lunch: Vietnamese Shirataki Soup (1.5 g)
Dinner: Herbal Green Beans and Chicken (4 g)
Snack or Dessert: Walnut Cookies (1.1 g)

Day 9:
Breakfast: Mexican Breakfast Casserole – Crockpot (5.2 g)
Lunch: Asian Style Zucchini Salad (7 g)
Dinner: Roasted Leg of Lamb (1 g)
Snack or Dessert: Zucchini Spiced Cupcakes (3.5 g)

Day 10:
Breakfast: Cinnamon Walnut Flax Muffins (2 g)
Lunch: Black Bean Quiche (5.1 g)
Dinner: Chicken Enchilada Bowl (6.14 g)
Snack or Dessert: Cocoa Butter Walnut Fat Bombs (0.3 g)

Day 11:
Breakfast: Oven-Baked Pancake With Bacon and Onions (5 g)
Lunch: Caprese Salad (4.58 g)
Dinner: Bacon Burger and Cabbage Stir Fry (4.5 g)
Snack or Dessert: Walnut Cookies (1.1 g)

Day 12:
Breakfast: Breakfast Meal-Prep Bombs (2.7 g)
Lunch: Cauliflower and Shrimp Salad (5 g)
Dinner: Beef and Broccoli - Slow Cooked (3 g)
Snack or Dessert: Pumpkin Cheesecake (4 g)

Day 13:
Breakfast: Cream Cheese Coffee Cake (4.2 g)
Lunch: Loaded Chicken Salad (6.74 g)
Dinner: Miso Salmon (0.78 g)

Snack or Dessert: Peanut Butter Cups (2 g)

Day 14:
Breakfast: Brunch Mackerel and Egg (Plate for Brunch (4 g)
Lunch: Egg Drop Soup (3 g)
Dinner: Pan-Glazed Chicken and Basil (4.6 g)
Snack or Dessert: Baked Apples (16 g)

Day 15:
Breakfast: Maple Pumpkin Flaxseed Muffins (2 g)
Lunch: Steak Salad (1.5 g)
Dinner: Pork Carnitas - Instant Pot (1 g)
Snack or Dessert: Blueberry Cream Cheese Bombs (1.02 g)

Day 16:
Breakfast: Maple Cinnamon 'Noatmeal' (4.4 g)
Lunch: White Chicken Chili (4 g)
Dinner: Lemon and Dill Wild-Caught Salmon - Slow-Cooked (2 g)
Snack or Dessert: Chocolate Chip Cheesecake Fat Bombs (1 g)

Day 17:
Breakfast: Bacon Hash (9 g)
Lunch: Grilled Buffalo Chicken Lettuce Wraps (2 g)
Dinner: Slow-Cooked Steak Tacos (4 g)
Snack or Dessert: Lemon Cheesecake Fat Bombs (0.5 g)

Day 18:
Breakfast: Cheesy Ham and Chive Soufflé (5 g)
Lunch: Broccoli Cheddar Soup (2 g)
Dinner: Stuffed Meatloaf (1.42 g)

Snack or Dessert: Orange and Walnut Chocolate Fat Bombs (2 g)

Day 19:
Breakfast: Single-Serve Baked Eggs (0.6 g)
Lunch: Lemon Garlic Shrimp Pasta (3.5 g)
Dinner: Grilled Chicken With Spinach and Mozzarella (3.7 g)
Snack or Dessert: Guacamole Deviled Eggs (5 g)

Day 20:
Breakfast: Sausage Egg Muffin (3.5 g)
Lunch: Feta Cheese Salad With Balsamic Butter (8 g)
Dinner: Grilled Pork Kebabs (3.3 g)
Snack or Dessert: Chocolate Dipped Candied Bacon (1.1 g)

Day 21:
Breakfast: Strawberry Donuts (0.6 g)
Lunch: Salad Sandwiches (3 g)
Dinner: Instant Pot Chicken Adobo (6.5 g)
Snack or Dessert: Blueberry Cupcakes (2.8 g)

Day 22:
Breakfast: Mexican Breakfast Casserole – Crockpot (5.2 g)
Lunch: Cauliflower and Mushroom Risotto (4.3 g)
Dinner: Asian Style Tuna Patties (3.8 g)
Snack or Dessert: Spicy Deviled Eggs (1 g)

Day 23:
Breakfast: Chocolate Pecan Pie and Muffins (3.4 g)
Lunch: Broccoli and Tuna (3 g)
Dinner: Cheeseburger Calzone (3 g)
Snack or Dessert: Chocolate Chip Cheesecake Fat Bombs (1 g)

Day 24:
Breakfast: Almost "McGriddle" Casserole (3 g)

Lunch: Beef and Cheddar Platter (6 g)
Dinner: Baked Tilapia and Cherry Tomatoes (4 g)
Snack or Dessert: Pumpkin Cheesecake (4 g)

Day 25:
Breakfast: Lemon Sour Cream Muffins (3 g)
Lunch: Halloumi Burger (9.4 g)
Dinner: Thai Green Chicken Curry – Instant Pot (5 g)
Snack or Dessert: Creamy Lime Pie (4.2 g)

Day 26:
Breakfast: Quiche Cups (2.1 g)
Lunch: Chicken Salad With Kiwi and Feta (13 g)
Dinner: Ginger and Sesame Salmon (2.5 g)
Snack or Dessert: Bacon Guacamole Fat Bombs (1.4 g)

Day 27:
Breakfast: Maple Cinnamon 'Noatmeal' (4.4 g)
Lunch: Chicken Sausage Corn Dogs (4.5 g)
Dinner: Barbacoa Beef (2 g)
Snack or Dessert: Chocolate-Filled Peanut Butter Cookies (2.7 g)

Day 28:
Breakfast: Egg Muffins - Six-Pack (1.1 g)
Lunch: Cauliflower and Shrimp Salad (5 g)
Dinner: Baked Whole Turkey (1 g)
Snack or Dessert: Apple Crisp With Blackberries (13 g)

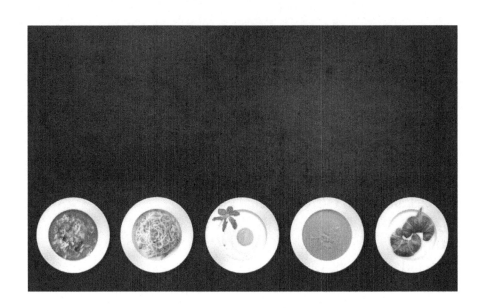

Chapter 9: A Final Word

You are almost there; just continue following your meal plan guidelines and add your favorites for your next round of intermittent fasting.

Mindset and Potential - Follow the Golden Rules

Remain Consistent During Fasting: Regardless of the type of weight loss that you ultimately choose to pursue, it is essential to pick one and stick with it. Attempting an intermittent fast for a few days before switching to another plan such as the Paleo diet before trying out a low-carb approach will only cause your body to freak out and hold on to every possible calorie until it figures out what in the world is happening.

Remember, fasting regularly and consistently is the surest way to see any of its benefits. Only after your body has time to adjust to your new routine will it then be able to adapt appropriately. It can begin to increase the number of positive enzymes and neural pathways to maximize weight loss using this method. Consider consistency in the ace-in-the-hole of proactive weight loss success.

Maintain Your Self-Control: Intermittent fasting only works if your body goes entirely without food for at least twelve hours; any caloric intake resets the cycle. As such, it is imperative to ensure that you maintain control of your bodily urges if you hope to see real results from this type of approach. Remember, fasting for at least twelve hours will only allow you to eat as you usually would or slightly more than an average meal. It does not give you a license to eat everything in sight. Keeping your appetites in check is a strict requirement for success.

Maintain a calorie Deficit: While this is true for any diet, it is even more true for intermittent fasting since it can be so easy to overeat once you do eat in such a way that it negates any benefits you might have felt. Remember, on average, you need to burn 3,500 calories weekly to lose one pound each week.

Eliminate all you can eat buffets. This is a nightmare for portion control. Don't tempt fate if you're just beginning your new diet program. Choose a smaller plate when you go to the buffet. You can also choose a normal size plate or fill it half full of veggies or salad.

Consider using free apps to assist you in if your goal is focused on weight loss. You have made the right choice using the Mediterranean Diet, so let's go one step further:

- *MyFitnessPal* has been chosen as one of the best apps available to track your macros. It's free to download, but you can also choose to update to a premium plan for higher rates.

- *My Food Diary* will provide you with the nutritional facts to ensure you have the correct carbohydrates, protein, and fats in your diet plan.

Use Supplemental Spices

Even with the batch of new recipes you now have; you might want to adventure on your own. These are a few spices to assist your solo preparation:

Black Pepper: Pepper promotes nutrient absorption in the tissues all over your body, speeds up your metabolism, and improves digestion. The main ingredient of pepper is a pipeline which gives it the pungent taste. It can boost fat metabolism by as much as 8%

for up to several hours after it's ingested. As you will see, it is used throughout your healthy Mediterranean recipes.

Cayenne Pepper: The secret ingredient in cayenne is capsaicin, which is a natural compound to give the peppers the fiery heat. This provides a short increase in your metabolism. The peppers are also rich in vitamins, effective as an appetite controller, smooths out digestion issues, and benefit your heart health.

Nutmeg: You will enhance your foods with the warm, slightly nutty flavor of nutmeg as it is often used in desserts and curries. The nutmeg seeds are compounds that act as antioxidants in your body. It also carries anti-inflammatory properties to assist in adverse health conditions such as arthritis, diabetes, and heart disease. Also noteworthy is its ability to protect with harmful bacteria, including Streptococcus mutans and E. coli, with its beneficial antibacterial components.

Cinnamon: Use cinnamon as part of your daily plan to improve your insulin receptor activity. Just put one-half of a teaspoon of cinnamon into a smoothie, shake, or any other dessert.

Cloves: Cloves possess a spicy yet sweet flavor, but also contain powerful natural medicine including strong antiseptic and germicidal components that can help ward off arthritis pain, gum and tooth pain, infections, and also relieve digestive problems.

Raw Ginger Root involves over 25 antioxidants. It maintains hefty anti-inflammatory elements to help reduce muscle aches and the pain and swelling of arthritis. Ginger is best known for its ability to reduce nausea and vomiting and with its soothing remedy for sore throats from outbreaks of flu and colds. Have a tea made with hot water simmered with a small amount of lemon and honey and a few slices of ginger as a soothing tonic at times when you're sick.

Basil: You can use fresh or dried basil to maximize its benefits. Its dark green color is an indication it also maintains an outstanding source of magnesium, calcium, and vitamin K, which is excellent for your bones. It also helps with allergies, arthritis or inflammatory bowel
conditions.

Cumin Powder: Cumin maintains abundant antioxidants which are excellent for your <u>digestion</u> and so much more. It also stimulates the pancreas and gallbladder to secrete bile and enzymes which work to break down the food into usable nutrients your body needs to function healthily. Cumin also helps detoxify the body and is beneficial for several respiratory disorders, including bronchitis and asthma. Cumin is also an excellent source of vitamin A and C as well as iron, which are all excellent for your immune system.

Downsides of Intermittent Fasting

For Women: Ask yourself these questions to discover whether any of the intermittent plans will help you:

- Do you want to become pregnant?
- Are you pregnant?
- Have you ever suffered from eating disorders – such as anorexia?
- Do you have diabetes?
- Do you have hypoglycemia?
- Are you underweight?

Clue: Each answer should be 'no' for you to be a suitable candidate for the diet technique. If you said 'yes' to them, it is definitely not the time to start the program.

These are further indications:

Children: Until a child reaches his/her 18th birthday, fasting is not advisable. They are still growing and require more nutrients daily.

Thyroid and Adrenal Issues: Proceed with caution because individuals with either of these problems have issues when dealing with stress. Fasting has been perceived as exacerbating the pre-existing condition.

Type 1 Diabetics: Your blood sugar naturally drops when fasting. If you are on insulin-lowering drugs, you will need to consult your physician before beginning the fasting process. It is possible for you to lower the dosage during your dieting.

PossibleBowel Issues: The biggest one of these is the initial change in your bowel movements as periods of constipation or in some cases, diarrhea could occur. Fortunately, they should not last more than a few days as your body adjusts to the new method of caloric intake.

Additional damage can be done to the body if periods of fasting are routinely followed by periods of excessive binging. It is vital to attempt intermittent fasting, and your periods of eating after, in moderation. If you notice any immediate severe physical changes after you begin any form of dieting regime, it is essential for you to consult a nutritionist or your physician.

Lastly, these are all precautions and may not have an effect on your experience. Please enjoy your new lifestyle changes on the way to becoming healthier.

Conclusion

I hope you better understand how to drop those unwanted pounds and become healthier with your personal copy of *Intermittent Fasting and Keto Diet: Smart Guide for Weight Loss, Heal your body and Live a Healthier Life; Includes Intermittent Fasting for Women and 28-Day Meal Plan With Quick and Delicious Keto Recipes*, let's hope it was informative and able to provide you with all of the tools you need to achieve your goals whatever they may be.

Staying busy is essential to combating food or drink cravings once you begin any new dieting techniques. You need to remove the *craving* from your head, so you can break the hold it has on you. Try one or all of these suggestions. Organize your computer files. That could take a while if you are like most individuals.

Write in a journal about your health goals. Catch up on your favorite hobby or start one like drawing or painting to keep your hands and mind occupied. Look through some photo albums to break a smile. Call a friend and talk about anything that does not pertain to food or drinks. These are just a few of the things you can do to break the craving chain, but you get the idea.

Walk away with the knowledge learned and prepare a feast using your delicious new recipes and meal plan. Be the envy of the neighborhood when you provide a feast at the next neighborhood gathering. Show off your skills and be proud. You can also boast of how much better you feel using the ketogenic diet plan.

Finally, if you found this book useful in any way, a review on Amazon is always appreciated!

Index for the Recipes

- Cauliflower and Shrimp Salad
- Chicken Salad With Kiwi and Feta
- Feta Cheese Salad With Balsamic Butter
- Loaded Cauliflower Bowl
- Loaded Chicken Salad
- Salad Sandwiches
- Shrimp Avocado Salad With Tomatoes and Feta
- Steak Salad
- Swedish Dill Shrimp Salad

Soup and Chili

- Asiago Tomato Soup
- Broccoli Cheddar Soup
- Egg Drop Soup
- No Beans Beef Chili
- Vietnamese Shirataki Soup
- White Chicken Chili

Other Luncheon Favorites

- Bacon and Shrimp Risotto
- Beef and Cheddar Platter
- Black Bean Quiche
- Broccoli and Tuna
- Cauliflower and Mushroom Risotto
- Chicken Sausage Corn Dogs
- Grilled Buffalo Chicken Lettuce Wraps
- Halloumi Burger
- Lemon Garlic Shrimp Pasta

Chapter 5: Dinner Specialties

Chicken and Poultry Favorites

- Baked Whole Turkey
- Balsamic Chicken Thighs

- Chicken Enchilada Bowl
- Grilled Chicken With Spinach and Mozzarella
- Herbal Green Beans and Chicken
- Instant Pot Chicken Adobo
- Pan-Glazed Chicken and Basil
- Slow-Cooked Teriyaki
- Thai Green Chicken Curry - Instant Pot

Beef Options

- Bacon Burger and Cabbage Stir Fry
- Barbacoa Beef
- Beef and Broccoli - Slow Cooked
- Cheeseburger Calzone
- Cube Steak- Instant Pot
- Oven-Roasted Burgers
- Slow-Cooked Steak Tacos
- Stuffed Meatloaf
- Taco Cabbage Skillet

Pork and Lamb Options

- Grilled Pork Kebabs
- Pork Carnitas - Instant Pot
- Pork-Chop Fat Bombs
- Roasted Leg of Lamb

Seafood and Other Options

- Asian Style Tuna Patties
- Baked Tilapia and Cherry Tomatoes
- Ginger and Sesame Salmon
- Lemon and Dill Wild-Caught Salmon - Slow-Cooked
- Miso Salmon
- Zucchini Lasagna With Tofu Ricotta and Walnut Sauce

Bread Option: Dinner Rolls

Chapter 6: Scrumptious Desserts

- Apple Crisp With Blackberries
- Blueberry Cupcakes
- Chocolate-Filled Peanut Butter Cookies
- Creamy Lime Pie
- Dark Chocolate Milkshake
- Peanut Butter Cups
- Peanut Butter Pie
- Pecan Pie Clusters
- Pumpkin Cheesecake
- Walnut Cookies
- Zucchini Spiced Cupcakes

Fat Bombs

- Blueberry Cream Cheese Bombs
- Chocolate Chip Cheesecake Fat Bombs
- Cocoa Butter Walnut Fat Bombs
- Lemon Cheesecake Fat Bombs
- Orange and Walnut Chocolate Fat Bombs

Chapter 7: Healthy Snack Options

- Almond Coconut Bars
- Bacon Guacamole Fat Bombs
- Baked Apples
- Chocolate Dipped Candied Bacon
- Cinnamon Vanilla Protein Bites
- Guacamole Deviled Eggs
- Spicy Deviled Eggs

Made in the USA
Middletown, DE
16 January 2020